Springer Series on Geriatric Nursing

Mathy D. Mezey, RN, EdD, FAAN, Series Editor
New York University Division of Nursing

Ivo Abraham, PhD, RN, FAAN, is President of the Epsilon Group L.L.C., an international health care consulting group. He holds faculty appointments at the University of Virginia, Katholieke Universiteit Leuven (Leuven, Belgium), and New York University. Dr. Abraham has more than 15 years of experience in leading-edge and internationally recognized research-and-development work in health care experience in results-oriented consulting and advisory work on international perspectives on health care and health systems. He received his B.S. (equivalent) from the Katholieke Universiteit Leuven (Belgium), and M.S. and Ph.D. from the University of Michigan. He has authored over 200 publications in health care, information technology, and statistics.

Melissa Marie Bottrell, MPH, is director of the Nurses Improving Care to the Hospitalized Elderly (NICHE) project, at the John A. Hartford Institute for the Advancement of Geriatric Nursing Practice. As the project director, she works with nurses and institutions nationwide to assist them in improving their geriatric nursing practice. She is a PhD candidate in Bioethics and Public Policy and an Adjunct Professor at the Robert. F. Wagner Graduate School of Public Service at New York University. She received her Bachelor of Arts in Bioethics from Pomona College and her Masters of Public Health from Boston University. She has written on topics as diverse as geriatric nursing research, public health, and bioethics.

Terry Fulmer, RN, PhD, FAAN, is a Professor of Nursing at New York University Division of Nursing, Director of the NYU Center for Nursing Research and co-Director for The John A. Hartford Foundation Institute for the Advancement of Geriatric Nursing Practice, and Director of the Consortium of New York Geriatric Education Centers. She received her bachelor's degree from Skidmore College and her master's and doctoral degrees from Boston College. She has held hospital appointments at the Beth Israel Hospital in Boston and the Yale-New Haven and NYU Medical Centers. Dr. Fulmer's research focuses on acute care of the elderly and specifically, the subject of elder abuse. Her books *Inadequate Care of the Elderly: Health Care Perspective on Abuse and Neglect,* and *Critical Care Nursing of the Elderly* (Springer Publishing Company) have received the *American Journal of Nursing* Book-of-the-Year Awards.

Mathy Doval Mezey, RN, EdD, FAAN, received her undergraduate and graduate education at Columbia University. She was a professor at the University of Pennsylvania School of Nursing, and Director of the Robert Wood Johnson Foundation Teaching Nursing Home Program, a national initiative to link schools of nursing and nursing homes. Currently, Dr. Mezey is a professor at New York University in the Division of Nursing, where she holds a Chair as the Independence Foundation Professor of Nursing Education and directs the Hartford Institute for the Advancement of Geriatric Nursing Practice. The focus of the Hartford Institute is to improve care received by older adults by stimulating best practices in nursing education, clinical care, research, and public policy. Dr. Mezey has authored 5 books and has over 50 publications that focus on nursing care of the elderly and bioethical issues that effect decisions at the end of life. Her research focuses on improving nursing care to older adults, and she is involved in several studies that explore how best to improve decision making about life-sustaining treatment.

Geriatric Nursing Protocols for Best Practice

Ivo Abraham, PhD, RN, FAAN
Melissa M. Bottrell, MPH
Terry Fulmer, PhD, RN, FAAN
Mathy D. Mezey, EdD, RN, FAAN
Editors

 Springer Publishing Company

Copyright © 1999 by Springer Publishing Company, Inc.

Springer Publishing Company, Inc.
536 Broadway
New York, NY   10012-3955

Cover design by Janet Joachim
Acquisitions Editor: Ruth Chasek
Production Editor: Pam Lankas

99 00 01 02 03 / 5 4 3 2 1

Library of Congress Cataloging-in-Publication Data

Geriatric nursing protocols for best practice / Ivo Abraham
   ... [et al.], editors.
      p.   cm. — (Springer series on geriatric nursing)
   Includes bibliographical references and index.
   ISBN 0-8261-1251-X (hardcover)
      1. Geriatric nursing.   2. Aged—Diseases—Nursing.   3. Aged—Care.
   I. Abraham, Ivo   II. Series: Springer series on geriatric
   nursing (Unnumbered)
      [DNLM: 1. Geriatric Nursing.   2. Nursing Assessment.
   3. Hospitalization—in old age.   WY 152 G3698 1999]
   RC954.G465   1999
   610.73'65—dc21
   DNLM/DLC
   for Library of Congress   98-52113
                                                                 CIP

Printed in the United States of America

CONTENTS

FOREWORD

We are entering an era in which people who require hospitalization are increasingly old and ill. Nursing and medical staff experienced in steering patients safely through surgery and/or recovery from a single medical illness often find themselves overwhelmed by the number and types of conditions with which many of these elderly patients present.

To be sure, most older people sail through a hospitalization without serious or lasting complications. Most improve further after discharge. But for many others, hospitalization is a "sentinel event," triggering a downward trajectory in health and function that is permanent. The negative consequences of a hospitalization are particularly noticeable in already frail older persons: those who already have compromised function, multiple chronic illnesses, and/or cognitive impairments.

We know quite a lot about the events that can turn a routine hospitalization into a cascade of negative outcomes for older people. These events include delirium, pressure ulcers, falls, and altered sleep patterns. We know quite a lot about what triggers these events, including excessive use of physical restraints; inappropriate drugs, dosages and duration of medications; inappropriate treatment of pain; and failure to address nutritional needs of older people.

Geriatric nurses and geriatricians have long recognized that negative outcomes are not inevitable consequences of a hospital-ization. Quite the contrary, careful assessment and planning can avert or minimize many complications. Over the past 15 years, a series of careful demonstration projects have taught us much about how to provide optimum care for the elderly in hospitals. One of the most prominent of these efforts, funded by The John A. Hart-ford Foundation, was The Hospital Outcomes Program for the Elderly (HOPE). HOPE projects were instrumental in demonstrat-ing the benefits of such service reconfigurations as units special-ized in the care of older people (Acute Care of the Elderly [ACE] units)[1], and of unit-based Geriatric Resource Nurses working with geriatric nurse specialists and geriatricians[2,3].

Yet despite these and other projects, the infusion of knowledge as to how to create a safer hospital environment for older people has been slow to take hold. It is to address this need that the editors have prepared this book of protocols. The protocols were specifically designed for the inpatient setting. Each represents a distillation of what constitutes "best practice" for 14 clinical syn-dromes that are commonly experienced by older people in hospi-tals. Already tested by nurses in eight hospitals, we are confident that these protocols address many of the needs of the practicing nurse at the bedside.

The protocols that appear in this book reflect the efforts of many authors and practicing nurses. We hope that they will prove useful in your setting and that they will directly benefit the older people who come under your care. We are confident that your use of these approaches and feedback to the authors will lead to new, "best practice" in geriatrics. These in turn will improve the qual-ity, outcomes, and cost-effectiveness of inpatient care. Today's and tomorrow's patients, their families or other caregivers, and their health practitioners will all be the beneficiaries of such changes.

DONNA REGENSTREIF, PHD
Senior Program Officer
The John A. Hartford Foundation of New York City

REFERENCES

[1] Landefeld, CS, Palmer, RM, Kresevic, DM, Fortinsky, R, Kowal, J. A randomized trial of care in a hospital medical unit especially designed to improve the functional outcomes of acutely ill older patients. *N Engl J Med.* 1995;32:1333-1338.

[2] Fulmer, T. Grow your own experts in hospital elder care. *Geriatr Nurs.* 1991;12:64-66.

[3] Inouye, SK, Acampora, D, Miller, RL, Fulmer, T, Hurst, LD, Cooney, LM. The Yale Geriatric Care Program: A model of care to prevent functional decline in hospitalized elderly patients. *J Am Geriatr Soc.* 1993;41:1345-1352.

PREFACE

The delivery of quality care during the acute, ever-shortening episode for the hospitalized elderly has become a major concern to families, staff nurses, nursing leadership, the chief nursing executive, medical staff, risk managers, and finance leaders alike. The percentage of the population that is aging is steadily, predictably rising, and the average age of members of this group is similarly rising. The multiplicity of problems imposed by each episode of hospitalization for the older patient proliferates. Their care needs are posing more complex challenges to nursing staff in particular, because frequently the problems requiring superb application of the nursing process are not disease specific, and are not generally amenable to standard medical regimens.

Although most organizations and health care systems have at least the rudiments of standards of practice for care, which focus on the process of care for specific patient groups, the development of such standards is a daunting project for the nursing staff. These nurses must be supported in their quest for methods and means of improving care delivery. Therefore, the focus of practice protocols is the staff nurse, the key critical element in the older person's survival in the institutional setting, or in the provider-supported program at home, as many elderly are supported in varying forms of home care services.

The purpose of this text is to present a compilation of geriatric nursing protocols that have been developed as part of involvement in the NICHE Project, or Nurses Improving Care to the Hospitalized Elderly. The 14 care problems commonly presented by sick elders to challenge staff nurses serve as the topic headings. The practice protocols each follow the conceptual framework of the professional nursing process: assessment of factors, specialized tools specific to the problem area if developed, care approaches and interventions, and evaluation of expected outcomes. Each protocol is research or evidence-based, thus providing the critical foundation of knowledge that has been tested.

This text serves many audiences, each of whom may be invested in some aspect of geriatric care: For the staff nurse at the bedside, these ready-to-use protocols provide a sound and sophisticated basis for the delivery and improvement of care. For resource nurses, nursing leadership, clinical specialists, case managers, and staff development instructors, these protocols provide substance and resources for either the development or modification of whatever standards model the organization has established. Administrators and educators in health care organizations seeking ideas and a rationale for age-specific features, now a critical element in Joint Commission on Accreditation of Health Care Organizations standards, will find that the basis for competency assessments tailored to the care of the elderly in this volume. Patient-care-quality-and-improvement experts will find that the content and tools provide clinically appropriate avenues for designing or enhancing programs establishing baseline parameters and desired outcomes to be achieved.

For students, this volume provides a role model for the breadth of thinking and application of knowledge required for advanced nursing practice. For the very educated public, these protocols pose the means by which to evaluate the practice level of the institution in which family members or significant others are actual or potential patients. For administrators of insurance plans, these protocols provide a professional nursing care-based means of determining the level of service that optimally should be provided.

The reader must be cautioned that the presentation of such process standards does not ensure their implementation. This collection serves, however, as a substantive foundation for the identification of the problems posed, research-based assessment and interventions, and evaluation of outcomes.

Susan Bower-Ferres, PhD, RN, CNAA
Vice President for Nursing Senior Administrator
NYU Medical Center

CONTRIBUTORS

Karen Allen, MS, RN
Former Graduate Student
University of Massachusetts
Amherst, MA

Elaine Jensen Amella, PhD, RN, CS, GNP
Assistant Professor
College of Nursing
University of Arizona
Tucson, AZ

Christine Bradway, MSN, RN, CS
University of Pennsylvania
Philadelphia, PA

Roberta L. Campbell, MSN, RN
Research Project Manager, PhD Student
University of Pennsylvania
Division of Nursing
Orexel, PA

Barbara Corrigan, MS, RN, CS
Geriatric Clinical Nurse Specialist
Baystate Medical Center
Springfield, MA

Kathleen Fletcher, RN, CS, MSN, GNP
University of Virginia Health and Sciences Center Clinician
Charlottesville, VA

Marquis D. Foreman, PhD, RN, FAAN
Associate Professor, College of Nursing
University of Illinois at Chicago
Chicago, IL

Deborah Francis, RN, CS, MS
Geriatric Nurse Clinician
University of California
Sacramento, CA

Sharon Hernley, MS, GNP
Suncity West, AZ

Denise M. Kresevic, PhD, RN, C
Geriatric Clinical Nurse Specialist
University Hospitals of Cleveland, Ohio
Cleveland, OH

Lenore H. Kurlowicz, PhD, RN, CS
Psychiatric Consultation Liaison Nurse
Hospital of the University of Pennsylvania
Philadelphia, PA

Lorraine C. Mion, RN, PhD
Director of Nursing Research
Cleveland Clinic Foundation
Cleveland, OH

Janet Moore, MS, RN, CS
Research Assistant
Baystate Medical Center
Springfield, MA

Mary D. Naylor, PhD, RN, FAAN
University of Pennsylvania
Associate Dean
School of Nursing & Director of Undergraduate Studies
Philadelphia, PA

Gloria Ramsey, RN, BSN, JD
Director, Legal & Ethical Aspects of Practice
New York University
School of Education
Division of Nursing
New York, NY

Patricia Samra, MS, RN
Former Graduate Student
University of Massachusetts
Amherst, MA

Cheryl Stetler, PhD, RN, FAAN
Specialist for Evidence-Based Practice
Baystate Medical Center
Springfield, MA

Neville Strumpf, PhD, RN
Associate Professor
University of Pennsylvania
Division of Nursing
Philadelphia, PA

Joyce Thielen, MS, RN, CS
Research Assistant
Baystate Medical Center
Springfield, MA

Lark J. Trygstad, RN, MA-ARNP-C
Internal Medicine
Mason City, IA

Mary K. Walker, PhD, RN, FAAN
Associate Professor
University of Kentucky
College of Nursing
Tampa, FL

May L. Wykle, PhD, RN, FAAN
Professor
Francis Payne Bolton School of Nursing
Case Western Reserve University
Cleveland, OH

INTRODUCTION

Mathy Mezey and Terry Fulmer

There is mounting evidence that we are reaching a crisis in caring for patients who require a hospital stay. Because many of the conditions that used to require a hospital stay are treated on an outpatient basis, and because patients in the hospital are moved quickly into stepped-down levels of care, only the very sick are now cared for in hospitals. Many of the patients have multiple diseases that further complicate their hospital stay. The overwhelming majority of patients are 65 years of age and over, and have the added burden of age-related changes that further complicate their hospitalization and impede their recovery.

It is paramount, then, that hospital nurses have at their fingertips tools that allow them to appropriately care for these elderly patients. Developed by nursing experts around the country as part of the Nurses Improving Care to the Hospitalized Elderly (NICHE) project, the 14 clinical protocols contained in this book are meant to serve as these tools. The goal of NICHE, initially funded by The John A. Hartford Foundation Inc., is to provide practicing nurses with the expertise to care for elderly patients who require hospitalization.

More generally, the NICHE Project is a national initiative to assist hospitals to position themselves to meet the needs of acutely ill elders. In conjunction with a team of nationally recognized leaders in geriatric nursing and tested in over 30 institutions around the country, NICHE has created a variety of tools to help facilities *assess* the perceptions of their staff regarding the quality of care they currently provide to elders, *modify* nursing care practice to better meet elders needs, and *evaluate* the effectiveness of those interventions. The NICHE Tools include the following:

- The *Geriatric institutional Assessment Profile* (GIAP), which is designed to assess attitudes regarding care of the elderly, nursing knowledge of institutional guidelines for care of the elderly, nursing knowledge of common geriatric syndromes, and perceived institutional barriers to best nursing practice for elders;
- *Nursing care models* that help reorganize nursing care to more efficiently and effectively meet the special needs of acutely ill elders;
- Research-based *clinical-practice protocols* reflect "best nursing practices" on 14 important geriatric syndromes including use of physical restraints, preventing pressure ulcers, sleep disturbances, advance directives, pain management and assessing cognitive function;
- Clinical and institutional *outcome indicators*, that match the clinical parameters in the GIAP and can be used to evaluate the effectiveness of the implementation of the nursing-care models and clinical-practice protocols; and
- A *consumer survey*, which captures the opinions of patients and families regarding the quality of clinical care provided to hospitalized elders.

Using NICHE, hospitals sites have improved geriatric care along a number of different parameters. The knowledge of nurses and other staff regarding "best practice" in care of the elderly has increased and along with it staff attitudes towards elders have improved. Further, sites have seen shorter hospital stays, reductions in urinary-tract infections, decreased severity and incidence of delirium, and reductions in iatrogenic complications.

As part of the work of the NICHE project to provide practicing nurses with the tools and expertise necessary to care for older adults, the protocols in this book represent "best practice" as it is currently recognized.

They reflect current research and nationally promulgated standards, including those developed by The Agency For Health Care Policy Research (AHCPR). On the other hand, the protocols are "user-friendly," in that they have been adapted to fit the exigencies of the nurse practicing in today's hospital. The protocols are meant to help the practicing nurse prevent, recognize, treat, and refer clinical conditions that they encounter frequently in caring for elderly medical and surgical patients. In using the protocols, we hope that nurses will feel more confident in the care that they provide their elderly patients, and more satisfied with their practice.

The 14 topics were chosen because they represent the key clinical conditions and circumstances likely to be encountered by a hospital nurse caring for older adults. The protocols are designed to be used and integrated into clinical practice either exactly as they are, or modified to fit the specific issues of an institution's patient population or unit parameters. Most of the protocols have been implemented in hospitals, both large and small, around the country. Although the protocols were developed for the acute care setting, the protocol's structure, which includes background, assessment parameters, care strategies, and evaluation for expected outcomes, allows the protocols to be modified to work in other practice settings, such as the nursing home or home care, or to be implemented by nurses at a variety of skill levels and license types.

Because we recognize that protocol development in no way assures protocol implementation, we have included a chapter on implementation to help institutions translate clinical knowledge into actual practice.

We have many people to thank for this book. We want to thank the many NICHE faculty members for their expertise and commitment. Neither these protocols nor the NICHE project would have been possible without the inordinate amount of work contributed by these individuals. We would also like to thank the institutions who supported the work of our authors. Without their foresight and commitment to older adults, these protocols would not have been developed.

THE NICHE FACULTY

Ivo Abraham, PhD, RN, FAAN, Principal and Managing Director, The Epsilon Group LLC, Charlottesville, VA

Elaine Jensen Amella, PhD, RN, CS, Assistant Professor, Medical University of South Carolina, Charleston, SC

Christine Bradway, MSN, RN, CS, Division of Nursing, University of Pennsylvania, PA

Melissa Bottrell, MPH, Project Director, Division of Nursing, New York University, New York, NY

Barbara Corrigan, MS, RN, CS, Geriatric Clinical Nurse Specialist, Baystate Medical Center, MA

Kim Dash, MPH, Educational Development Center Inc, Newton, MA

Priscilla Ebersole, PhD, RN, FAAN, Professor Emeritus, San Francisco State University, San Francisco, CA

Kathleen Fletcher, RN, CS, MSN, GNP, Clinician, University of Virginia Health and Sciences Center, Charlottesville, VA

Marquis Foreman, PhD, RN, FAAN, Associate Professor and Clinical Scientist, College of Nursing, University of Illinois at Chicago, Chicago, IL

Deborah Francis, RN, CS, MS, Geriatric Clinical Specialist, University of California, Davis Medical Center

Terry Fulmer, PhD, RN, FAAN, Professor, Division of Nursing, New York University, New York, NY

Denise Kresevic, PhD, RN, C, Geriatric Clinical Nurse Specialist, University Hospitals of Cleveland, Cleveland, OH

Lenore Kurlowicz, PhD, RN, CS, Psychiatric Consultation Liaison Nurse, Hospital of the University of Pennsylvania, PA

Mathy Mezey, RN, EdD, FAAN, Professor, Division of Nursing, New York University, New York, NY

Loraine Mion, RN, PhD, Senior Nurse Researcher, Cleveland Clinic Research Foundation, Cleveland, OH

Mary D. Naylor, PhD, RN, FAAN, Associate Dean and Director of Undergraduate Studies, School of Nursing, University of Pennsylvania, PA

Gloria D. Ramsey, RN, JD, Director of Legal and Ethical Aspects of Practice, Division of Nursing, New York University, New York, NY

Neville Strumpf, PhD, RN, Associate Professor, Division of Nursing, University of Pennsylvania, PA

Lark J. Trygstad, RN, MA-ARNP-C, Geriatric Nurse Practitioner, North Iowa Mercy Health Center, Mason City, IA

Cheryl Vince-Whitman, EdM, Vice President, Education Development Center, Inc, Newton, MA.

Mary K. Walker, PhD, RN, FAAN, Professor, University of South Florida College of Nursing, Tampa, FL

May L. Wykle, PhD, RN, FAAN, Professor, Francis Payne Bolton School of Nursing, Case Western Reserve University, Cleveland, OH

Chapter 1

ASSESSMENT OF FUNCTION: CRITICALLY IMPORTANT TO ACUTE CARE OF ELDERS

Denise M. Kresevic, Mathy Mezey, and the NICHE Faculty

EDUCATIONAL OBJECTIVES

On completion of this article, the reader should be able to:
1. Discuss perceptions of hearing loss by nursing home residents.
2. Describe nursing activities to assist persons with hearing loss.
3. Discuss the concept of functional decline.

Twenty to forty percent of all elders experience functional decline during hospitalization[1]. Risk factors for functional decline include injuries, acute illness, medication side effects, depression, malnutrition, and decreased mobility, including the use of physical restraints and iatrogenic complications[2]. Assessment of function by acute care nurses is especially important. In one randomized clinical trial of hospitalized elders, the daily nursing assessment of ability to perform bathing, dressing, grooming, toilet-

Reproduced from Kresevic, DM, Mezey, M. Assessment of function: Critically important to acute care of elders. *Geriatric Nursing*, 1997, *18*, 216–222. With permission from Mosby-Year Book, Inc.

TABLE 1.1   Functional Assessment of Elders

Dimension	Assessment Parameter	Standardized Instrument	Nursing Strategies
ADL			
Bathing	Self-report of	Katz ADI[3]	Encourage active
Dressing	patient, family		participation in
Eating	or Home Nurse	ADL Situation	ADLs and assist as
Toileting		Test[17]	needed
Hygiene	Direct observation	Functional	Orient to unfamiliar
Transferring	while in the	Status[18]	environment
	hospital		Encourage to be out of bed
		Performance	Ambulate daily
		Test of	Consult with PT/OT
		ADL[19]	for strengthening
			exercises and adaptive
			equipment
Mobility			
Transferring	Self-report of		Transferring
	patient, family		Encourage active and
	or Home Nurse		passive range of motion
	regarding some		Encourage and assist out
	and frequency		of bed ambulation
	of performance		
Walking	Observe:	Get Up and	Walking
	Balance	Go Test[17]	Physical therapy
consult			
	Gait		for exercises and
	Distance		equipment
	Capacity		Referral to community
			exercise programs
			Referral for visual testing
IADL			
Housework	Direct observation	Lawton	Community resources for
Accounting		IADL[16]	housework/accounting
Transportation	Self-report of	Medication	Transportation
Medications	patient, family or	Management	Vision screening
	Home Nurse	Test[20]	
Food	Simulated		Identify community
preparation	evaluation, e.g.		Home meals
Shopping	evaluation by OT		Transportation
	for kitchen		Pharmacy delivery
	safety		Pill counters

ing, transferring, and ambulation during routine nursing care yielded information necessary for maintenance of function in self-care activities[1].

Nurses are in a pivotal position in all care settings to assess elders' functional status by direct observation during routine care and through information gathered from the elder, the family, and long-term caregivers. Systematic functional assessment in the acute care setting can provide a *benchmark* of patients' progress as they move along the continuum from acute care to rehabilitation or from acute to subacute care. The ongoing use of a standardized functional assessment instrument promotes systematic communication of patients' health status between care settings and allows units to compare their level of care with other units in the facility and to measure outcomes of care (Table 1.1). This article addresses the goals of and need for functional assessment of elderly individuals in acute care and provides a clinical practice protocol to guide nurses in the functional assessment of elderly individuals. (Table 1.2).

ASSESSMENT TECHNIQUES AND ASSESSMENT PARAMETERS

Functional assessments are constantly conducted by nurses every time they notice that a patient can no longer pick up a fork or has difficulty walking. A comprehensive functional assessment leads to more than simply noticing a change in activity or ability, however. In a systematic manner, nurses need to assess the ability of a patient to perform activities of daily living (ADLs) in context of the patient's baseline functional status and hospitalization status. Any decrease in functional status should prompt an immediate search for underlying causes.

A variety of instruments/methods are available for conducting functional assessments including the Katz ADL Index[3], the Barthel (instrumental activities of daily living [IADL]) index[4,5] and the Older American Resources and Services (OARS) assessment[6–8]. The Katz ADL index has been the most widely used in a variety of settings. It has established reliability and is easy to

TABLE 1.2   Nursing Standard of Practice Protocol: Assessment of Function in Acute Care

The following nursing care protocol has been designed to assist bedside nurses to monitor function in elders, prevent decline, and to maintain the function of elders during acute hospitilization.

Objective: The goal of nursing care is to maximize the physical functioning and prevent or minimize decline in ADL function.

I. Background
    A. Functional status of individuals describes the capacity to safely perform ADL. Functional status is a sensitive indicator of health or illness in elders and therefore a critical nursing assessment.
    B. Some functional decline may be prevented or ameliorated with prompt and aggressive nursing intervention (e.g. ambulation, enhanced communication, adaptive equipment).
    C. Some functional decline may occur progressively and is not reversible. This decline often accompanies chronic and terminal disease states such as Parkinson's Disease and dementia.
    D. Functional status is influenced by physiological aging changes, acute and chronic illness, and adaptation. Functional decline is often the initial symptom of acute illness such as infections (pneumonia, urinary tract infection). These declines are usually reversible.
    E. Functional status is contingent on cognition and sensory capacity including vision and hearing.
    F. Risk factors for functional decline include injuries, acute illness, medication side effects, depression, malnutrition, and decreased mobility (including the use of physical restraints).
    G. Additional complications of functional decline include loss of independence, socialization, and increased risk for long-term institutionalization and depression.
    H. Recovery of function can also be a measure of return to health such as those individuals recovering from exacerbations of cardiovascular disease.
II. Assessment Parameters
    A. A comprehensive functional assessment of elders includes independent performance of basic ADL, social activities, or IADL, the assistance needed to *accomplish* these tasks, and the sensory ability, cognition, and capacity to ambulate.
        1. Basic ADL
            a. Bathing
            b. Dressing
            c. Grooming
            d. Eating
            e. Continence
            f. Transferring

(continued)

TABLE 1.2 *(continued)*

2. Instrumental activities of daily living
   a. Meal preparation
   b. Shopping
   c. Medication administration
   d. Housework
   e. Transportation
   f. Accounting
B. Elderly patients may view their health in terms of how well they can function rather than in terms of disease alone.
C. The clinician should document functional status and recent or progressive declines in function.
D. Function should be assessed over time to validate capacity, decline, or progress.
E. Standard instruments selected to assess function should be efficient to administer, easy to interpret, and provide useful practical information for clinicians.
F. Multidisciplinary team conferences should be scheduled.

III. Care Strategies
A. Strategies to maximize function
   1. Maintain individual's daily routine. Assist to maintain physical, cognitive, and social function through physical activity and socialization. Encourage ambulation, allow flexible visitation including pets, and reading the newspaper.
   2. Educate elders and caregivers on the value of independent functioning and the consequences of functional decline.
      a. Physiological and psychological value of independent functioning
      b. Reversible functional decline associated with acute illness
      c. Strategies to prevent functional decline. Exercise, nutrition and socialization
      d. Sources of assistance to manage decline
   3. Encourage activity including routine exercise, range of motion, and ambulation to maintain activity, flexibility, and function.
   4. Minimize bed rest.
   5. Explore alternatives to physical restraints use.
   6. Judiciously use psychoactive medications in geriatric dosages.
   7. Design environments with hand rails, wide doorways, raised toilet seats, shower seats, enhanced lighting, low beds, and chairs.
   8. Help individuals regain baseline function after acute illnesses by using exercise, physical therapy consultation, and increasing nutrition.
   9. Obtain assessment for physical and occupational therapies needed to help regain function.
B. Strategies to help individuals cope with functional decline
   1. Help elders and family determine realistic functional capacity with interdisciplinary consult.

(continued)

TABLE 1.2   *(continued)*

    2. Provide caregiver education and support for families of individuals when decline cannot be ameliorated in spite of nursing and rehabilitative efforts.

    3. Carefully document all intervention strategies and patient responses.

    4. Provide information to caregivers on causes of functional decline related to the patient's disorder.

    5. Provide education to address safety care needs for falls, injuries, and common complication. Alternative care settings may be required to ensure safety.

    6. Provide sufficient protein and caloric intake to ensure adequate intake and prevent further decline.

    7. Provide caregiver support community services, such as home care, nursing, and physical and occupational therapy services, to manage functional decline.

IV. Expected outcomes

  A. Patients can

    1. Maintain safe level of ADL and ambulation.

    2. Make necessary adaptations to maintain safety and independence including assistive devices and environmental adaptations.

  B. Provider can demonstrate

    1. Increased assessment, identification, and management of patients susceptible to or experiencing functional decline.

    2. Ongoing documentation of capacity, interventions, goals, and outcomes.

    3. Competence in preventative and restorative strategies for function.

  C. Institution can demonstrate

    1. Incidence and prevalence of functional decline will decrease in all care settings.

    2. Decrease in morbidity and mortality rates associated with functional decline.

    3. Decreased use of physical restraints.

    4. Decreased incidence of delirium.

    5. Increase in prevalence of patients who leave hospital with baseline functional status.

    6. Decreased readmission rate.

    7. Increased utilization of rehabilitative services (occupational and physical therapy).

    8. Support of institutional policies/programs that promote function.

      a. Caregiver educational efforts

      b. Walking programs

      c. Continence programs

      d. Self-feeding initiatives

      e. Elder group activities

use, gathering information by observation on bathing, dressing, eating, transferring, continence, and grooming. Elders are evaluated according to levels of independence. The Barthel Index for physical functioning includes bathing, grooming, continence, stair climbing, and the ability to propel a wheelchair. This instrument has been useful in rehabilitation settings to monitor improvements over time. The Barthel instrument allows differentiation among task performance, including amount of help and amount of time needed to accomplish each task. The OARS instrument for physical function is similar in scope of measurement to the Katz scale, including bathing, dressing, grooming, and continence. However, unlike the Katz instrument, which uses caregiver observation, the OARS relies on self-report. Self-reports of capacity may be less valid than observations of performance, with some elders overestimating or underestimating actual capacity[9]. Further, the "Get Up and Go Test" actually assesses performance of ambulation (See Box 1). The assessment of IADL, including ability to prepare meals and administer medications safely, may not be observed during an acute hospitalization, although assessment of capacity in these domains has important implications for planning for posthospitalization services. Regardless of the instrument used, basic ADL function should be assessed for each patient including capacity for dressing, eating, transferring, toileting, hygiene, and ambulation. Appropriate assessment instruments should be readily available on acute care units. To adequately assess function, sensory capacity and cognitive capacity must be established.

Ambulation

The ability to walk is a critical parameter for functional assessment. Some instruments used to assess ambulation, balance, and gait are sensitive measures of mobility[10]; however, they are also complex and time consuming to use. Instruments such as "The Get Up and Go" test[11] yield valuable information on independence in ambulation with efficiency and ease of use. Direct observation of an individual's ability to get out of bed, sit in a chair, assume a standing position, and steadily walk a short distance with or without assistive devices is important to ensure safety in

BOX 1.   The "Get Up and Go" Test For Gait Assessment in Elderly Patients

Have the patient sit in a straight-backed high-seat chair
Instructions for patient:
  Get up (without use of armrests, if possible)
  Stand still momentarily
  Walk forward 10 ft (3 m)
  Turn around and walk back to chair
  Turn and be seated
Factors to note:
  Sitting balance
  Transfers from sitting to standing
  Pace and stability of walking
  Ability to turn without staggering

From Mathias, Nayak, and Isaacs[11].

to ADL capacity[10,11]. Direct observation of transfer and ambulation should include an assessment of speed of performance, hesitancy, stumbling, swaying, grabbing for support, or unsafe maneuvers such as sitting too close to the edges of a chair or dizziness while pivoting[12]. The *Get Up and Go* test (Box 1) for gait assessment is one tool that can be easily used by nurses for ambulation assessments in older individuals[10]. Assessment of unsafe transfers or ambulation indicates the need to begin immediate restorative therapies to prevent injuries and falls.

Sensory Capacity

Evaluation of the potential impact of sensory issues on the performance of ADLs is often overlooked. A simple test for functional vision is to have elders read a headline or sentence from the newspaper. A moderate impairment can be noted if only the headline can be read[12]. If the elder has eyeglasses, they must be available and cleaned.

Hearing ability is essential to function and cognition. Individuals with decreased hearing may be inaccurately labeled as cognitively impaired. Hearing aides may not have been sent to the hospital with the elder. These may be obtained by the family. Beside hearing acuity may be validated by asking patients to identify the sound of a ticking watch. The "whisper test" may also be used. This is done by whispering 10 words while standing 6 inches away from the individual. Inability to repeat five of the words indicates a need for further assessment of hearing acuity. Visualization of the external ear canal by cerumen may identify one easily treatable problem in decreased hearing acuity, however[13]. Individuals with hearing deficits detected as part of bedside assessment should be referred for additional assessment and treatment including hearing aides. Headphone amplifier devices may be a useful and inexpensive item to stock on nursing units in hospitals.

Cognitive Capacity

Cognitive function is a major factor in a person's functional capacity. Baseline function is important to assess. However, such assessments most often initially rely on information provided by family members because acute illnesses may be clinically manifested as acute confusional states[2]. Components of cognitive function, including attention, language, and memory can be assessed by nurses during interviews and routine care, although anxiety and illness may be complicating factors. Fluctuating attention may indicate acute reversible impairment or temporary reactions to hospitalization. Foreman et al. give guidelines for cognitive assessment in a clinical practice protocol; see chapter 6 in this book[15].

Cause

All instances of functional decline should be assessed for cause. Patients experiencing any acute loss of ADL independence should be thoroughly assessed for acute illness. In the presence of acute illness, such as urinary tract infection, pneumonia, or recovery after surgery, impaired independent ADLs are expected to return to baseline with appropriate care and rehabilitation as the illness resolves. Comprehensive musculoskeletal or neurologic examination, laboratory tests, or referral for a therapeutic trial of physical or occupational therapy may be needed.

USE OF ASSESSMENT INFORMATION

Nursing care during the acute phase of illness is aimed at encouraging elders to get out of bed for meals, to perform bathing and dressing activities, and to participate in occupational and physical therapy to avoid iatrogenically induced decline and prevent additional complications. Individuals for whom an acute illness is superimposed on chronic conditions, such as arthritis or Parkinson's disease, may need aggressive strategies to maintain their level of independence and to prevent unnecessary deterioration in ADL. Early referral to occupational and physical therapy for the purpose of prescriptive activities and assessment of IADLs must not be neglected.

An assessment of selected instrumental activities of daily living including shopping, housework, finances, food preparation, medication administration, and transportation must be part of comprehensive discharge planning[16]. In summary, for older people, evaluation of function represents the cornerstone of good nursing care and affords a sound baseline by which to provide information essential to plan for continued care across settings.

A CASE STUDY

Mrs. Brown*, a 93–year-old widow, was admitted to a general medical surgical nursing unit after her daughter found her at home, clothing in disarray and mumbling incoherently. A chest Xray in the ER revealed pneumonia, and her blood work revealed severe dehydration, with an elevated serum sodium and blood urea nitrogen. Mrs. Brown's daughter assured the nursing staff that her mother had been living alone independently and caring for her own physical needs such as bathing, dressing, and eating before this episode of illness.

As soon as Mrs. Brown arrived on the unit, she began screaming for her daughter. In spite of attempts to assist Mrs. Brown to walk, she was unable to take more than one or two steps before she froze in place. The nursing staff, fearful of a fall, used a vest

---

*Pseudonym

restraint to keep Mrs. Brown in the chair. She developed incontinence and refused food and fluids, in spite of efforts by the nurse
aide to feed her. She continued to scream for her daughter all
evening. The night nurse convinced the physician on call to order
haloperidol (Haldol) 5 mg stat for agitation. Rather than mitigat-
ing or reducing Mrs. Brown's agitation, it escalated throughout
the night. Exhausted, she fell asleep in the early morning hours.

The next day Mrs. Brown's daughter arrived with her mother's
glasses, hearing aid, and walker. That afternoon, with her glasses
and hearing aid on, Mrs. Brown began to ask what had happened
to her. She drank two glasses of juice and ate a bowl of chicken
soup. Using her wheeled walker she was able to ambulate independently to the bathroom and even to the nurses station to find
a newspaper. An early comprehensive assessment and history
taking that included contact with her daughter might have prevented the fear, confusion, and agitation Mrs. Brown experienced
on her first day of hospitalization.

ACKNOWLEDGMENT

Supported by a grant from the John A. Hartford Foundation.

REFERENCES

[1] Landefeld SC, Palmer RM, Kresevic DM, Fortinsky RH, Kowal J. A
    randomized trial of care in a hospital medical unit especially de-
    signed to improve the functional outcomes of acutely ill older pa-
    tients. *N Engl J Med.* 1995;332:1338–44.
[2] Creditor MC. Hazards of hospitalization of the elderly. *Ann Intern
    Med.* 1993;118:219–223.
[3] Katz S, Ford AB, Moscokowitz RW, Jackson BA, Jaffe MW. Studies of
    illness and the aged: The index of ADL. A standardized measure of
    biological and psychosocial function. *JAMA.* 1963;185: 914–919.
[4] Mezey MD, Rauckhorst LH, Stokes SA. *Health Assessment of the Older
    Individual.* New York: Springer Publishing;1993.
[5] Mahoney FL, Barthel DW. Functional evaluation: the Barthel index.
    Maryland State Med J. 1965;14: 61–65.

[6] Burton RM, Damon, WW, Dillinger DC, Erickson DJ, Peterson DW. Nursing home rest and care: An investigation of alternatives. In: Pfeiffer E, Ed. *Multidimensional Functional Assessment: The DARS Methodology.* Durham, NC: Duke Center for Study of Aging Human Development; 1978.

[7] Kane RA, Kane RL. *Assessing the Elderly: A Practical Guide to Measurement.* Lexington, MA: Lexington Books; 1988.

[8] Applegate WB, Blass J, Franklin T. Instruments for the functional assessment of older patients. *N Engl J Med.* 1990;322:1207–1214.

[9] Cress ME, Schectman KB, Mulrow CD, Fiatarone MA, Gerety MB, Buchner DM. Relationship between physical performance and self-perceived physical function. *J Am Geriatr Soc.* 1995;43:93–101.

[10] Tinetti ME, Ginter SF. Identify mobility dysfunctions in elderly patients: standard neuromuscular examination or direct assessment? *JAMA.* 1988;259:1190–1193.

[11] Mathias S, Nayak US, Isaacs B. Balance in elderly patients: The "Get Up and Go" test. *Arch Phys Med Rehab.* 1986;67:387–389.

[12] Trueblood PR, Rubenstein LZ. Assessment of instability and gait in elderly persons. *Compr Ther.* 1991;17:20–29.

[13] Abrams WB, Berkow R, Eds. *The Merck Manual of Geriatrics.* White House Station, NJ. Merck, Sharp & Dohme Research Laboratories;1990.

[14] Woolf SH. Screening for hearing impairment. In: Goldbloom RB, Lawrence RS, Eds. *Preventing Disease: Beyond the Rhetoric.* New York: Springer-Verlag; 1990:331–346.

[15] Foreman MD, Fletcher K, Mion LC, Simon L. *Assessing Cognitive Function.* Geriatric Nursing 1996;17:228–233.

[16] Lawton MP, Brody EM. Assessment of older people: Self-maintaining and instrumental activities of daily living. *Gerontologist.* 1969;9:179–186.

[17] Skurla E, Rogers JC, Sunderland T. Direct assessment of activities of daily living in Alzheimer's disease: A controlled study. *J Am Geriatr Soc.* 1988;36:97–103.

[18] Lowenstein DA, Amigo E, Duara R, Guterman A, Hurwitz D, Berkowitz N, et al. A new scale for the assessment of functional status in Alzheimer's Disease and related disorders. *J Gerontol.* 1989;44:114–121.

[19] Kurianski J, Gurland B. The performance test of activities of daily living. *Int J Aging Human Dev.* 1976;7:343–352.

[20] Gurland BJ, Cross P, Chen C, Wilder DE, Pine ZM, Lantigua RA, Fulmer T. A new performance test of adaptive cognitive functioning: the medication management (MM) test. *Int J Geriatr Psychiatr.* 1994;9:875–85.

Chapter 2

SLEEP DISTURBANCES IN ELDERLY PATIENTS

Marquis D. Foreman, May Wykle, and the NICHE Faculty

EDUCATIONAL OBJECTIVES

On completion of this chapter, the reader should be able to:
1. Define several causes of alterations in the sleep–wake cycle.
2. Identify factors that place older patients at risk for alterations in the sleep-wake cycle.
3. Identify the consequences of sleep disturbances in hospitalized older patients.
4. Describe parameters for a comprehensive sleep assessment.
5. Plan nonpharmacologic and individualized strategies for dealing with sleep disturbances in hospitalized older patients.

Sleep is a mechanism for restoring the body and its function and maintaining energy and health[1]. It has a renewing and replenishing effect, both physically and emotionally. Sleep is a necessity for survival[2]. When sleep is disrupted, physical, emotional, and behavioral disturbances arise. With severe disruption of sleep,

Reproduced from Foreman, M., Wykle, M. Nursing standard-of-practice protocol: Sleep disturbances in elderly patients. *Geriatric Nursing,* 1995, *16,* 238–243. With permission from Mosby-Year Book, Inc.

physiologic instability may occur. Thus, for everyone, adequate sleep is essential. It is particularly essential for older adults who are receiving medical care. This chapter presents a nursing standard of practice protocol for sleep disturbances in elderly patients. Foundational to this nursing standard of practice is a discussion of sleep, the changes in sleep that accompany aging, and an overview of sleep disorders.

REM AND NREM

Sleep, a complex combination of physiologic and behavioral processes, is defined as "a reversible behavioral state of perceptual disengagement from and unresponsiveness to the environment[3]." Within sleep, there are two states: Rapid eye movement (REM), or desynchronized, sleep and nonrapid eye movement (NREM), or synchronized, sleep[3].

NREM sleep accounts for approximately 75% to 80% of total sleep time and is characterized by a minimum of mental activity in a movable body[3]. REM sleep, entered some 60 to 90 minutes into the sleep cycle, accounts for about 20% to 25% of total sleep time and is considered essential for well-being[2]. REM sleep, characterized by an abundance of mental activity, as reflected by electroencephalographic activation, and rapid eye movements, is associated with dreaming. In REM sleep there is muscle atonia; blood pressure, pulse, and respiration increases and fluctuates[2]. Deprivation of REM sleep is associated with anxiety, irritability, inability to concentrate, and, if the deprivation is severe enough, disturbed behavior[2,4].

The sleep cycle usually progresses from stage-1 NREM sleep, through stages 2, 3, and 4, to REM sleep. REM sleep typically occurs after a change from stage-3 or stage-4 NREM to stage-2 NREM sleep, and continues to alternate between REM and NREM stages in 70-to 120–minute cycles. Typically there are 4 to 6 cycles per night. According to Carskadon and Dement[3], during the first third of a typical night, stages 3 and 4 NREM sleep predominate, while in the last third, stage-2 NREM and REM sleep predominate and stage-4 NREM sleep may be absent.

TABLE 2.1   Common Changes in Sleep with Aging

- Decrease in actual time asleep
- Increase in total sleep time (i.e., more time in bed but less of it asleep)
- Increase in sleep latency (i.e., more time required to fall asleep)
- Increase in the number of awakenings each night
- REM sleep more interrupted
- Increase in stage 1 sleep
- Stages 3 and 4 sleep less deep
- Decreased sleep efficiency
- More easily disturbed by environmental factors
- More frequent comments about poor quality of sleep
- Increase in daytime sleepiness and napping

CHANGES IN SLEEP WITH AGING

Changes in the way people sleep as they age occur as with other human mechanisms[5]. The changes in sleep observed with aging are listed in Table 2.1; these changes lead to sleep that is lighter, shorter, and interrupted. These changes are for the most part minor, still allowing for sleep to achieve its restorative function. Recent evidence indicates that changes observed in sleep are more likely to be the result of chronic health problems and their treatment than of aging[6,7]. However, elders are predisposed to poor sleep as a result of heightened autonomic activity and an increased susceptibility to external arousal[6]. In addition to these normal changes in sleep that accompany aging, there are disturbances in the sleep–wake cycle that are not normal.

These alterations in sleep require prompt and appropriate assessment and intervention, as they are associated with increased morbidity, mortality, and a reduction in the quality of life[1,4,5]. These alterations in the sleep–wake cycle have been classified into four major categories, summarized in Table 2.2: (1) dyssomnias, (2) parasomnias, (3) sleep disorders associated with medical or psychiatric disorders, and (4) proposed sleep disorders[8,9]. Each category is described in the text that follows.

Dyssomnias are disorders of initiating and maintaining sleep (also known as *insomnias*) and those of excessive somnolence[8,9]. The dyssomnias are the primary sleep disorders associated with disturbed nighttime sleep and impaired wakefulness[8,9]. These

TABLE 2.2   The International Classification of Sleep Disorders

Dyssomnias
  Intrinsic sleep disorders, e.g., Narcolepsy, Nocturnal myoclonus
  Extrinsic sleep disorders, e.g., Environmental sleep disorder, Hypnotic
    dependent sleep disorder
  Circadian rhythm sleep disorders, e.g., Time-zone change (jet lag) sleep
    disorder, Shift-work sleep disorder

Parasomnias
  Arousal disorders, e.g., Confusional arousals, Sleepwalking
  Sleep–wake transition disorder, e.g., Rhythmic movement disorders
  Parasomnias associated with REM sleep, e.g., Nightmares
  Other parasomnias, e.g., Sleep enuresis, Primary snoring

Medical or Psychiatric Disorders
  Mental disorders, e.g., Psychoses, Mood disorders
  Neurologic disorders, e.g., Dementia, Parkinsonism
  Other medical disorders, e.g., Chronic obstructive pulmonary disease,
    Nocturnal cardiac ischemia

Proposed Sleep Disorders
  Menstrual-associated sleep disorder

Adapted from Thorpy[8] and Diagnostic Classification Steering Committee[9]
© 1990; American Sleep Disorders Association and the Sleep Research Society, Rochester, MN. Reprinted by permission.

dyssomnias are further divided into three major groups, based, in part, on pathophysiologic mechanisms: (1) intrinsic sleep disorders, (2) extrinsic sleep disorders, and (3) circadian rhythm sleep disorders. Intrinsic sleep disorders are disorders associated with complaints of insomnia or excessive sleepiness that are caused by processes within the body. Examples of intrinsic sleep disorders include narcolepsy, sleep apnea syndromes, and noctural myoclonus. Conversely, extrinsic sleep disorders are caused by processes external to the body, most frequently environmental in nature. Extrinsic sleep disorders also are characterized by insomnia and excessive sleepiness. Examples include disturbances in sleep resulting from excessive lighting or noise, caffeinated beverages, and hypnotic drug or alcohol dependence[8,9]. Circadian rhythm sleep disorders share a common chronobiologic etiology, and include: jet-lag syndrome, shift-work sleep disorder, and irregular sleep–wake pattern. Treatment of these disorders consists primarily of identifying the underlying pathophysiologic process and correcting, eliminating, or minimizing it.

Parasomnias are manifested by central nervous system changes, autonomic nervous system changes, and skeletal muscle activity[8,9]. They are disorders of arousal, partial arousal, and sleep-stage transition, caused not by abnormalities in basic sleep processes but by undesirable physical phenomena that occur during sleep[8–12]. Parasomnias are further subdivided into (1) arousal disorders, disorders associated with impaired arousal from sleep; (2) sleep–wake transition disorders, those that occur during the transition from sleep tp wakefulness or in sleep stage transitions; (3) parasomnias associated with REM sleep; and (4) other parasomnias[8,9]. Sleep–wake transition disorders are an exception in that they are considered to be caused by altered physiologic processes rather than by pathophysiologic changes[8,9].

Medical–psychiatric sleep disorders are those disturbances in sleep and wakefulness associated with a large number of health problems and their treatment. This category is further subdivided into three groups; these sleep disorders are associated with (1) mental, (2) neurologic, and (3) medical disorders. These disturbances in sleep, referred to by some as secondary sleep problems, are frequent concomitants of hospitalization for acute illness in older patients and may be remedied by a variety of nursing strategies. These sleep disorders, although common, are associated with poorer outcomes of hospitalization (delayed healing, protracted recuperation, transient states of cognitive impairment, and physiologic instability). Sleep disturbances also are associated with a decreased ability to function and to perform daily activities; therefore, these disturbances occasionally result in institutionalization. Despite these negative consequences of sleep disturbances, the sleep of hospitalized patients generally is not carefully assessed by nurses; interventions are predominately pharmacologically based and are more likely to exacerbate the sleep disturbance they were intended to solve (Table 2.3). The practice protocol in Box 1 outlines the parameters for the assessment of sleep and the nursing strategies for the prevention and management of sleep disturbances. Central to this practice protocol is the principle that

TABLE 2.3 **Drugs and Sleep Disturbances**

Drug type	Specific drug	Effect on sleep
CNS Depressants		
Barbiturates	Phenobarbital Nembutal Seconal	Suppresses REM sleep
Narcotics	Demerol	Suppresses REM sleep
Benzodiazepines	Valium Librium Dalmane Restoril Halcion Ativan Serax	Alters REM sleep; reverses normal sleep patterns
Alcohol		Reduces REM sleep and inhibits movement
CNS Stimulants	Caffeine Amphetamine Theophylline	Delays onset of sleep; interferes with REM sleep
Antipsychotics	Mellaril Haldol Thorazine Navane	Causes daytime drowsiness
Autonomic agents	Nasal sprays cough syrups with dextro- methorphan OTCs: Sudafed	Causes daytime sleepiness
Antihypertensives	Methyldopa Reserpine Atenolol Nifedipine	Causes drowsiness
Monamine oxidase inhibitors	Marplan Nardel Parnate	Improves sleep in depressed persons
Diauretics		Nighttime awakenings caused by nocturia
Steroids		Interferes with sleep

Adapted from Ebersole and Hess[2].

pharmacologically based interventions should be used as a temporary means of last resort. Parameters for the evaluation of these nursing strategies also are included.

Proposed sleep disorders is a category for newly described sleep disorders and those for which there is insufficient or inadequate information[8]. Information for establishing the nature of these sleep disorders is anticipated.

ASSESSMENT OF SLEEP

The underlying causes of sleep disturbances in the elderly population include acute and chronic illness and their treatment, characteristics of the hospital environment, characteristics of the older individual, and disruptions in daily routines. As a result, assessment of sleep and sleep disturbances should encompass the parameter of (1) usual sleep–wake patterns, (2) bedtime routines/rituals, (3) diet and drug use (not to overlook over-the-counter medications), (4) environmental factors, (5) physiologic factors, and (6) illness factors. Specific areas of questioning are found in the protocol for sleep disturbances in elderly patients. Information elicited should include objective data as well as subjective appraisals of the quality of sleep. Questions of family or significant others also may provide insight into usual patterns and certain aspects of sleep.

This assessment is focused to elicit information relative to indicators, or defining characteristics, of sleep disturbance, which include verbal comments by the individual of not sleeping well, of not feeling rested, of being tired, of being awakened earlier than usual, or of having interrupted sleep. Changes in behavior or performance also will be observed. For example, the person will be irritable, restless, lethargic, listless, or apathetic[13]. Additionally, the person may be observed to have difficulty concentrating, an increased reaction time, a greater sensitivity to pain, and diminished daytime alertness. If ambulatory, this person may be prone to accidents and falls.

NURSING STRATEGIES

Given the prevalence of sleep disturbances in older hospitalized patients and their association with poorer outcomes of care, it was clear to us that practice guidelines were needed. As part of the John A. Hartford Foundation's Nurses Improving Care of the Hospitalized Elderly (NICHE) Project, a panel of gerontologic nurse experts developed a standard of practice for hospital nurses to follow to prevent and manage sleep disturbances (see Box 1). This practice guideline for sleep was developed on two basic principles. First, for the strategy to be effective, it must be individualized, considering the specific characteristics of the patient and the nature of the sleep disturbance as determined by means of the sleep assessment. Second, pharmacologic treatment (e.g., prescription and administration of a sedative or hypnotic agent) should be considered an intervention of last resort. Additionally, when pharmacologic treatment is considered appropriate, only a short-acting, low-dose medication with a wide margin of safety is recommended on a temporary basis[14]. Nonpharmacologic strategies are emphasized in the protocol.

OUTCOMES/EVALUATION

Expected outcomes or the evaluation of the strategies selected should be based on the results of the assessment. Thus, if the selected strategies were successful, the indicators upon which the individual was determined to have a disturbance in sleep should be minimized or eliminated. For example, if the sleep disturbance was the result of interrupted sleep from a noisy environment, the appropriate strategy would be to reduce the frequency of interruptions to sleep and reduce the noise. Expected outcomes would include subjective verbalizations of having slept better or of feeling more rested. Objectively, there would be evidence of an increased ability to concentrate and a reduction of any previously observed behaviors related to sleep deprivation (e.g., restlessness). Evidence that the strategies are effective would include the observation of appropriate sleep periods (e.g., 6 to 8 hours per night),

Box 1. Nursing Standard of Practice Protocol: Sleep Disturbance in Elderly Patients

Assessment	Intervention	Evaluation
Sleep-wake patterns: • Inquire about usual times for retiring and rising, time for falling asleep; freq. and duration of nighttime awakenings; freq. and duration of daytime naps; daytime physical and social activity • Have person provide a subjective evaluation of the quality of sleep	Maintain normal sleep pattern: • Maintain usual bedtime • Schedule nighttime activities to provide uninterrupted periods of sleep of at least 2–3 hours • Balance daytime activity and rest • Discourage daytime naps • Promote social interaction	Objective evidence: • Time required to fall asleep; should fall asleep within 30–45 minutes • Time for awakening, at usual reported time • Observe duration of sleep; patient should remain asleep for at least 4-hour intervals
Bedtime routine/ritual: • Inquire about activities performed by the individual before bedtime (e.g., personal hygiene, prayer, reading, watching TV, listening to music, snacks)	Support bedtime routines/ rituals: • Offer a bedtime snack or beverage • Enable bedtime reading or listening to music • Assist with aspects of personal hygiene at bedtime (e.g., a bath) • Encourage prayer or meditation.	Subjective evidence: • Verbalizations about the quality and quantity of sleep, e.g., statements of difficulty falling asleep, frequent awakenings; having slept well, feeling well-rested/refreshed; of an increased sense of well-being
Medications: • Obtain information relative to all prescribed and self-selected over-the-counter medications used by person, especially, sleep-aids, diuretics, laxatives • Determine types of medications and length of time used by person	Avoid/minimize drugs that negatively influence sleep (see Table 2.3): • Pharmacologic treatment of sleep disturbances is treatment of last resort • Discontinue or adjust the dose or dosing schedule of any/all offending medications • Consider drug-drug potentiation • Administer meds to promote sleep; give diuretics at least 4 hours before bedtime	

(continued)

| Box 1. Nursing Standard of Practice Protocol (*continued*) |||
Assessment	Intervention	Evaluation
Diet effects: • Obtain information about the consumption of caffeinated and alcoholic beverages	Minimize/avoid foods that negatively influence sleep: • Discourage use of beverages containing stimulants (e.g., coffee, tea, sodas) in afternoon and evening • Encourage use of warm milk • Provide snacks according to patient preference • Generally discourage use of alcoholic beverages • Decrease fluid intake 2–4 hours before bedtime	
Environmental factors: • Evaluate noise, light, temperature, ventilation, bedding	Create optimal environment for sleep: • Keep noise to an absolute minimum • Set room temperature according to patient preference • Provide blankets as requested • Use night light as desired • Provide soft music or white noise to mask the noise of hospital activity	
Physiologic factors: • Evaluate breathing pattern with sleep, with attention to pauses • Observe for periodic movement or jerking during sleep • Inquire about usual position and the number of pillows used with sleep	Promote physiologic stability: • Elevate head of bed as required • Provide extra pillows per patient preference • Administer broncho-dilators, if prescribed, before bedtime • Use medical therapeutics (e.g., continuous positive airway pressure machine) as prescribed	*(continued)*

Box 1. Nursing Standard of Practice Protocol (*continued*)		
Assessment	Intervention	Evaluation
• Note diagnoses of sleep disorders (e.g., sleep apnea or narcolepsy) • Note diagnoses of specific health problems that adversely affect sleep (e.g., congestive heart failure)		
Illness factors: • Inquire about pain, affective disturbances (e.g., depression, anxiety, worry, fatigue, and discomfort)	Promote comfort: • Provide analgesia as needed 30 minutes before bedtime • Massage, back or foot, to help patient relax • Warm and cool compresses to painful areas as indicated • Assist with progressive relaxation or guided imagery • Encourage patient to urinate before going to bed • Keep path to bathroom clear or provide bedside commode	

(*continued*)

as well as an alert, attentive patient who is able to concentrate and who follows commands or directions.

Outcomes other than those that are patient-specific allow for a more precise evaluation of the quality of the care provided to older patients.

ACKNOWLEDGMENT

This protocol was developed as a part of the NICHE project, supported by a grant from the Hartford Foundation.

BIBLIOGRAPHY FOR DEVELOPMENT OF PROTOCOL

Jenike MA. *Geriatric Psychiatry and Psychopharmacology: A Clinical Ppproach*. St. Louis: Mosby-Year Book, 1989;272–88.

Johnson JE. Bedtime routines: Do they influence the sleep of elderly women? *J Appl Gerontol*. 1988;7:97–110.

National Institutes of Health. Treatment of sleep disorders of older people. *Consensus Statement*. 1990;8(3):1–22.

REFERENCES

[1] Spenceley SM. Sleep inquiry: a look with fresh eyes. *Image: J Nurs Sch*. 1993;25:249–56.

[2] Ebersole P, Hess P. Toward healthy aging: human needs and nursing response. 4th ed. St. Louis: Mosby; 1994:64–74.

[3] Carskadon MA, Dement WC. Normal human sleep: an overview. In: Kryger MH, Roth T, Dement WC, Eds. *Principles and practice of sleep medicine*. (2nd ed). Philadelphia: WB Saunders; 1994:16–25.

[4] Gottlieb GL. Sleep disorders and their management. *Am J Med*. 1990,88(suppl 3A):29S-33S.

[5] Prinz PN, Vitello MV, Raskind MA, Thorpy MJ. Geriatrics: Sleep disorders and aging. *N Engl J Med*. 1990;323:520–526.

[6] Bliwise DL. Normal aging. In: Kryger MH, Roth T, Dement WC, Eds. *Principles and Practice of Sleep Medicine.* 2nd ed. Philadelphia: WB Saunders; 1994:26–39.

[7] Beck-Little R, Weinrich SP. Assessment and management of sleep disorders in the elderly. *J Gerontol Nurs.* 1998;24:21–29.

[8] Thorpy MJ. Classification of sleep disorders. In: Kryger MH, Roth T, Dement WC, Eds. Principles and practice of sleep medicine. 2nd ed. Philadelphia: WB Saunders, 1994:426–36.

[9] Diagnostic Classification Steering Committee (Thorpy MJ, chairman). *International Classification of Sleep Disorders: Diagnostic and Coding Manual, revised.* Rochester, MN: American Sleep Disorders Association; 1997.

[10] Hayakawa T, Kamer Y, Vrata J, Shibui K, Osaki S, Uchiyama M, Okawa M. Trials of bright light exposure and melatonin administration in a patient with non-24 hr sleep–wake syndrome. *Psychiatry clin Neurosci.* 1998;52:261–262.

[11] Sedgwick PM. Disorders of the sleep–wake cycle in adults. *Posgrad Med J.* 1998;74:134–138.

[12] Brunner DP, Wirz-Justice A. Chronobiological sleep disorders and their treatment possibilities. *Ther Umsch.* 1993;50:704–708.

[13] Dudas S, Kim MJ. Sleep pattern disturbance. In: Kim MJ, McFarland GK, McLane AM, Eds. *Pocket Guide to Nursing Diagnosis.* (3rd ed). St. Louis: Mosby; 1989:258–261.

[14] Consensus Panel. Drugs and insomnia: the use of medications to promore sleep. *JAMA.* 1984;251:2410–2414.

_____Chapter **3**

EATING AND FEEDING DIFFICULTIES FOR OLDER PERSONS: ASSESSMENT AND MANAGEMENT

Elaine Jensen Amella and the NICHE Faculty

EDUCATIONAL OBJECTIVES

At the conclusion of this chapter, the reader will be able to:
1. Describe physiologic parameters used to assess the nutritional status of elderly patients.
2. Discuss the steps for a feeding assessment
3. Describe steps to maximize the social and cultural components of meals.
4. Describe ways that dementia may influence eating and feeding behaviors.

As individuals age, the likelihood of functional impairments increases. In the face of frailty and deconditioning, loss of function follows a predictable pattern with the ability to feed oneself the last activity of daily living (ADL) to be lost[1]. Numerous functional assessment instruments are based on this hierarchy of increased dependence. Interestingly, the ability to self-feed is the first ADL mastered as a child, and is the last ADL to be lost in old age. As with all activities, an individual's functional independence should be preserved. Therefore, self-feeding must be promoted for all persons for as long as possible.

Eating is the most social of all ADLs. Nutritional status is influenced by factors beyond the diet itself. Alterations in nutritional health may indicate unrecognized disease states or adverse reactions, unmet assistive needs, inattention to cultural norms, psychological problems, or lack of attention to the social aspects of dining. The professional nurse plays a critical role in recognizing and assessing problems with nutrition, eating, and feeding; implementing a plan of care that involves education and supervision of caregivers; and, appropriate referral to the interdisciplinary team .

RECOGNITION OF EATING AND FEEDING PROBLEMS

Existing instruments rate eating dependency as mild, moderate, or severe with no attempt to define areas of strength that may be amenable to intervention or maintenance[2]. Coexisting health problems that might compromise functioning, are rarely addressed, for example, vision loss or depression; preexisting social issues, such as food insecurity, the inability to purchase adequate food because of poverty; social isolation; or inattention to dining rituals. Thus, assessment of eating and feeding problems becomes like the proverbial story of the blind men describing the various parts of an elephant. An interdisciplinary team approach is critical, using specialized assessments with a case manager or professional nurse coordinating care.

For persons who have multiple sensory changes, cognitive losses, or well-established dining rituals, institutional mealtime routine may make food unacceptable and interfere with intake. For example, certain Muslims and Jews have strict requirements for preparation and blessing of food before it can be consumed. These elders may not eat rather than break dietary religious laws. Additionally, the use of the toilet and washing one's hands should be offered to all persons before meals.

The elder who may be in the terminal stages of illness should be consulted regarding personal wishes regarding food and fluid intake. When the elder loses the capacity for decision making, the proxy for health care decisions should be observed.

DIAGNOSIS AND MANAGEMENT OF EATING AND FEEDING PROBLEMS

History and Physical Assessment

For older persons, weight is considered the "Fifth Vital Sign," as so many health problems present initially with weight loss or gain. On admission, both height and weight are measured to calculate Body Mass Index (BMI), a much more sensitive indicator of nutritional problems that weight alone. Normal BMI for the elderly ranges from 22–27 and is calculated as weight in kg/height in meters-squared[3]. Height changes in the elderly. Therefore, height should be measured either standing or extrapolated from arm span or knee height [males: 64.19 (0.04 x age) + (2.02 x knee height); females: 84.88 – (0.24 x age) + (1.83 x knee height)][2].

The review of systems and physical examination focuses on key areas that influence eating and feeding. The nurse should pay particular attention to the need for adaptive equipment including eyeglasses, hearing aid, and special utensils needed to maintain independence. Oral health and hygiene are initially assessed and are included in ongoing assessments with preventative care or treatment by the dentist. Whenever possible, food should be maintained in its original form and not turned into a gruel. Pain should be routinely assessed and palliated. Problems with the gastrointestinal (GI) tract will compromise the desire to eat. Fatigue, illnesses, such as those involving the cardiopulmonary system, and certain treatments may make food less palatable[4].

Assessment of swallowing problems includes more than the simple gag reflex (test of Cranial Nerve X). Inattention to subtle signs that suggest choking may lead to patient aspiration[5]. All patients with known or suspected swallowing problems should be referred to the speech therapist. Videofluoroscopy is helpful in diagnosing swallowing disorders, however, the patient must be able to cooperate with the examination. Patients are assessed for proper sitting posture, upper body strength, fine and gross motor movement, and head and neck strength by the occupational therapist.

Medications may interact with food, altering absorption of key nutrients. Additionally, psychotropic and other neuroleptic drugs may negatively influence the patient's ability to eat, be fed, or safely ingest food. Tardive dyskinesia resulting from long-term use of psychotropics make it difficult to chew and swallow food. Consultation with a clinical pharmacologist is important.

Intake

The most accurate assessment of intake requires weighing and recording all food consumed. Using a food diary or calorie count confirms problems. The count should be conducted over a 3-day period with one of those days being on the weekend. Requesting the patient or family to assist in compiling the food diary will help emphasize the critical importance of eating. The registered dietitian should be involved in designing individualized intake records that can accurately assess the patient's intake. Within the institution, a 72-hour calorie count is routine. However, reports of estimated percentage of food consumed have been shown to be inaccurate in nursing homes[6].

Numerous biochemical parameters can be used to determine adequacy of nutritional intake. For elderly persons, laboratory diagnostics usually include: serum albumin, transferrin, hemoglobin, hematocrit, B_{12} levels, total cholesterol, and total lymphocyte count[7]. Low levels may indicate underlying pathology or malnutrition related to inadequate consumption of nutrients or undiagnosed wasting disorders[8].

Cognition

Discussion of the assessment and management of cognitive problems in the elderly has been reported in other NICHE protocols

Thorough neuropsychological testing can reveal problems in specific cognitive domains that may or may not be amenable to intervention. Many cognitive deficits impair the ability to eat.

In very late-stage dementia, persons may develop refuse-like or aversive behavior[9]. Watson[10] has developed a psychometrically sound instrument, the Ed-Fed, to measure the declining ability to consume food offered. Nurses can use the principles of this instrument to determine the stage of eating behavior. In the earlier stages, more active behaviors are displayed, for example, the individual pushes food away or turns the head away from the feeder. In later stages, passive behaviors occur, as the patient does not swallow and allows food to fall from the mouth. In late-stage dementia, a primitive and less forceful swallow pattern may develop. The upper airway is not well protected, making the use of bottle or syringe-type feeding not only undignified, but ineffective and unsafe.

Depression is one of the most common causes of weight loss in the elderly, and should be investigated in persons who manifest problems with eating or decline to be assisted with meals. Some medications prescribed for depression, for example, the selective serotonin reuptake inhibitors (SSRIs), may paradoxically depress the appetite in the elderly, while tricyclic antidepressants may potentiate appetite. Additionally, failure to thrive (FTT), a diagnosis once reserved for children, is now recognized as a major factor in frailty and weight loss in older persons[8]. Very frail persons may not have the physiologic reserve to feed themselves due to sacropenia (muscle wasting).

Environment/Ambience

Because of the strong social and cultural components of eating, where one dines is sometimes as important as what one eats. Simply, staff should ask themselves, "Would I want to eat my next meal where the patient is eating?" If the answer is "no," then steps should be taken to improve the dining area.

Small changes in the dining environment may make large improvements in the patient's capacity and motivation to eat or be fed[11]. Use of flatware and china plates, cups and saucers help to cue the patient. Removal of dishes from the tray and placing them directly on either a tablecloth or a placemat of contrasting or darker color provides visual cues as well as establishing the food as the patient's own. When the caregiver places the tray in front of him or herself and then reaches across to give the food to the patient, the patient may interpret this as eating from another person's plate.

In addition to avoiding medicalization of the eating space, the nurse should be alert for all the possible interruptions and disruptions that occur during the patient's meal. The number of interruptions during meals, even by persons walking in and out of the room, has been linked to lower intake[12]. When less than 50% of the meal is consumed, nurses should attempt to assess events surrounding that meal.

Relationship with Caregiver at Meals

Above all, dining is a shared experience. Successful completion of the meal is dependent on who assists or feeds the patient and the interpersonal process that person uses to interact with the patient[13,14]. Caregivers who are able to let the patient set the tempo of the meal and allow others to make choices will be more effectual. Unfortunately, time is a costly commodity within institutions. It is critical that the nurse, with the assistance of the speech therapist if the patient has swallowing problems, teach the family, friends, and nonprofessional caregivers how to safely assist the patient while preserving the patient's dignity and social aspects of the meal. These persons should be periodically supervised while assisting the patient. A volunteer program such as reported by Musson[15] may be helpful.

Touching and smiling have been correlated with improved intake[16]. Facing the patient on the same plane (*en face*) preserves the social aspects of dining and therefore may have esthetic value. Patients may need to be assisted into a functional eating posture or have assistive devices developed by the occupational or physical therapist to facilitate self-feeding[17].

Cuing is critical for patients with neuromuscular diseases or dementia. Whenever finger foods are given, they should be placed in the patient's hand. The caregiver may even assist by putting the patient's hand and arm through the motions a few times (hand-over-hand) while repeating simple cues. Pantomime of gestures assists to pattern the most effective eating strategies. Sitting more able patients next to the less able offers another opportunity for modeling appropriate behavior. Family-style dining (foods placed in serving dishes rather than on trays) offers an environmental context that is more akin to remembrances of meals past.

The patient should be allowed and encouraged to feed him or herself, to whatever degree possible. Adaptive equipment should be clean and readily available. Caregivers should be instructed in techniques that facilitate the social aspects of meals and set the stage for the task of eating, and should also be familiar with an individualized plan of care that fosters independence. The ideal model of practice is one that supports an individual in his or her attempts to eat independently for as long as possible[18]. See Table 3.1 (p. 35).

REFERENCES

[1] Katz S, Ford AB, Moskowitz, RW, Jackson BA, Jaffe MW. The index of ADL: A standardized measure of biological and psychological function. *JAMA*. 1963;185:915–919.

[2] Reuben DB, Greendale GA, Harrison GG. Nutrition screening in older persons. *J Am Geriatr Soc*. 1995;43:415–425.

[3] White J, Ham R, Lipschitz D. Consensus of the Nutrition Screening Initiative: Risk factors and indicators of poor nutritional status in older Americans. *J Am Dietet Assoc*. 991;91:783–787.

[4] Esberger K. Guide to gastrointestinal problems of elders. *Geriatr Nurs*. 1991;12:74–75.

[5] Amella EJ. Choking: Aspiration in the elderly. In C Bradway (Ed.), *Nursing Care of Geriatric Emergencies*. New York: Springer Publishing Company, 1996:154–169.

[6] Schell ES, Kayser-Jones J, Porter C. The recording of percentage of food eaten by nursing home residents: Fact or fiction? *Gerontol*. 1995;35(Special Issue 1):193–194.

[7] Barrocas A, Belcher D, Champagne D, Jastram C. Nutrition assessment practical approaches. *Clin Geriatr Med*. 1995;11:675–713.

[8]   Verdery R. Clinical evaluation of failure to thrive in older people. *Clin Geriatr Med.* 1997;13:769–778.

[9]   Norberg A, Backstrom A, Athlin E, Norberg B. Food refusal amongst nursing home patients as conceptualized by nurses' aids and enrolled nurses: An interview study. *J Adv Nurs.* 1988;13:478–483.

[10] Watson R. Measuring feeding difficulties in patients with dementia: perspectives and problems. *J Adv Nurs.* 1993;18: 25–31.

[11] VanOrt S, Phillips LR. Nursing interventions to promote functional feeding. *J Gerontol Nurs.* 1995;21(10):6–14.

[12] Deutekon EJ, Phillipsen H, Hoor TF, Abu-saad HH. Plate waste producing situations in nursing wards. *Int J Nurs Stud.* 1991;28:163–174.

[13] Amella EJ. Factors influencing the amount of food consumed by nursing home residents with dementia. *Gerontolo* 1996;36 (Special Issue 1):97.

[14] Athlin E, Norberg A, Asplund K, Jansson L. Feeding problems in severely demented patients seen from task and relationship aspects. *Scand J Caring Sci.* 1989;3:113–121.

[15] Musson ND, Frye GD, Nash M. Silver spoons: Supervised volunteers provide feeding of patients. *Geriatr Nurs.* 1997;18(1):18–20.

[16] Eaton M, Mitchell-Bonair IL, Freidman E. The effects of touch on nutritional intake of Chronic Brain Syndrome patients. *J Gerontol.* 1986;41:611–616.

[17] Ozer MN, Materson RS, Caplan LR. Management of Persons with Stroke. St. Louis, MO: Mosby Year Book; 1994.

[18] Osborn CL, Marshall M. Promoting mealtime independence. Geriatric Nursing 1992;18:254–256.

[19] Katz S, Downs TD, Cash HR, Grotz RC. Progress in the development of the Index of ADL. *Gerontol.* 1970;10:22.

[20] Siebens H, Trupe E, Siebens A, Cook F, Anshen S, Hanauer R, Oster G. Correlates and consequences of eating dependency in institutionalized elderly. *J Am Geriatr Soc.* 1986;34:193.

[21] American Psychiatric Association. Diagnostic and Statistical Manual of Mental Disorders (4th ed.) (DSM-IV). Washington, DC: Author; 1994:539.

[22] Morley JE. Anorexia of aging: physiologic and pathologic. *Am J Clin Nutr.* 1997;66:760–773.

TABLE 3.1   Protocol

Guiding principles:

1. The adequate intake of nutrients is necessary to maintain physical and emotional health.
2. Mealtime is not only an opportunity to ingest nutrients, but to maintain critical social aspects of life.
3. The social components of meals will be observed including mealtime rituals, cultural norms, and food preferences.
4. Persons will be encouraged and assisted to self-feed for as long as possible.
5. Persons dependent in eating will be fed with dignity.
6. End-of-life decisions by the individual or his or her proxy regarding the provision or termination of food and fluid will be respected.
7. The quality of mealtime is an indicator of the quality of life and care of an individual.

I. BACKGROUND
   A. Definitions:
      1. Feeding is "the process of getting the food from the plate to the mouth. It is a primitive sense without concern for social niceties[19].
      2. Eating is the "ability to transfer food from plate to stomach through the mouth" [20]. Eating involves: the ability to recognize food; the ability to transfer food to the mouth; and the phases of swallowing.
      3. Anorexia is "characterized by a refusal to maintain a minimally normal body weight"[21]. May have physiological basis in the elderly[8,22].
      4. Dysphagia is an impairment of the mechanisms of swallowing
      5. Apraxia is an inability to carry out voluntary muscular activities related to neuromuscular damage. As it relates to eating and feeding, loss of the voluntary stages of swallowing or the manipulation of eating utensils.
      6. Agnosia is the inability to recognize familiar items when sensory cuing is limited
   B. Etiology of problems with eating and feeding:
      1. Myopathies: Myasthenia gravis, sceloderma, congenital weakness, spasms of the esophagus;
      2. Neurogenic: Movement disorders especially Parkinson's Disease; ALS; dementia, especially Alzheimer's Disease; stroke with lesions of the upper motor neurons, brainstem, inferior portions of the precentral gyrus or the posterior portion of inferior frontal gyrus; cranial neuropathies related to cancer or diabetes;
      3. Systemic infections: Anorexia related to infections or sepsis;

(continued)

TABLE 3.1   *(continued)*

4. Mechanical disorders: Severe cervical spondylosis in C4 to C7 with osteophytes; tracheotomy tubes; significant kyphosis; poor dentition;
5. Psychological: Depression, anorexia, failure to thrive; or,
6. Iatrogenic: Adverse drug reactions especially tardive dyskinesia; poor or absent oral care; lack of adaptive equipment; untreated pain; use of physical restraints that limit ability to move, position, or self-feed; improper chair or table surface or discrepancy of chair to table height; use of wheelchair in lieu of table chair; use of disposable dinnerware especially for patients with cognitive or neuromuscular impairments.

II. ASSESSMENT
   A. Assessment with elder and caregivers
      1. Rituals used before meals, e.g., hand washing and toilet use. Dressing for dinner.
      2. Blessings of food or grace, if appropriate.
      3. Religious rites or prohibitions observed in preparation of food or before meal begins, e.g., Muslim, Jewish, Seventh Day Adventist. Consult with pastoral counselor, if available.
      4. Cultural or special cues—family history, especially rituals surrounding meals. Preferences as to end-of-life decisions regarding withdrawal or administration of food and fluid in the face of incapacity, or request of designated health-proxy. Ethicist or social worker may facilitate process.
   B. History and physical assessment (focused) coordinated with nursing and medicine.
      1. Weight and height—on admission to determine Body Mass Index (weight in kg/height in m2); thereafter weight taken at least every 7 days if a diagnosis of alteration in nutritional status exists.
      2. Skin—Lesions, turgor, dryness, hair loss.
      3. Neurological—Cranial nerves V, VII, IX, X, XI, XII (involved in swallowing).
      4. Sensory limitations—Vision, smell, taste, hearing.
      5. Oral cavity—Cleanliness, dentition including caries at root and surface, fit of denture or other oral appliances, lesions, condition of gums and tongue. Refer to Dentist for evaluation and treatment.
      6. Neck—Capacity to swallow. Refer to speech therapist for thorough assessment.
      7. Respiratory—Restrictive disease limiting ability to eat or tolerate larger quantities of food, exercise intolerance. Refer to respiratory therapist, if appropriate.
      8. Cardiac—Presence of congestive failure—Stages III or IV, or poorly controlled angina, indicating intolerance of any activity.

(continued)

TABLE 3.1 *(continued)*

9. GI—GERD, hiatal hernia, hypo- or hyperactive bowel (constipation or diarrhea), abdominal pain or tenderness, diverticular disease.
10. Strength and coordination—Neuro- and musculoskeletal exam, i.e., sitting posture, use of upper extremities including ROM, tremors, fine motor movements. Refer to occupational and physical therapist for assessment, as appropriate.
11. Psychological—Affective disorders, especially depression.
12. Pain—General and localized, especially in jaw, mouth, throat, GI.
13. Endocrine—Fasting blood sugar, microalbunemia and thyroid stimulating hormone in weight loss, for undiagnosed/poorly controlled diabetes and thyroid disease.
14. Medications—Sedation, abnormal movements. Pharmacologist to determine polypharmacy.

C. Intake (precise measurement needed as estimates can be inaccurate).
1. Calorie count for 3 days (including one weekend day, if in community).
2. Weighing of food (pre and post-meals, if precise intake is required).
3. Biochemical—Monitor laboratory diagnostics for abnormalities.
4. Diet history—Designed by registered dietitian and completed by nursing staff.

D. Cognition after diagnosis established through neuropsychological testing (use the 4 A's of Alzheimer's Disease as they influence eating, plus anorexia):
1. Aphasia—Can not verbally express preferences.
2. Apraxia—Can not manipulate utensils and food prior to eating, can not manipulate food within mouth/ swallow.
3. Agnosia—Can not recognize utensils, food.
4. Amnesia—Forgets having eaten, does not recognize need to eat.
5. Anorexia—Lack of desire to eat, possible physiological basis (FTT).

E. Environment/ambience:
1. Dining or patient room—Personal trappings versus institutional; no treatments or other activities occurring during meals; no distractions.
2. Tableware—Use of standard dinnerware, e.g., china, glasses, cup and saucer, flatware, tablecloth, napkin versus disposable tableware and "bibs."
3. Furniture—Elders seated in armed chair, table appropriate height versus eating in wheelchair or in bed.
4. Noise level—Environmental noise from music, caregivers, TV is minimal; personal conversation between patient and care giver is encouraged.

(continued)

TABLE 3.1 *(continued)*

    5. Light—Adequate and nonglare-producing versus dark, shadowy, or glaring.
    6. Odor—Familiar smells of food prepared versus all food prepared away from elder or medicinal smells and waste.
    7. Adaptive equipment—Available, appropriate, and clean; caregiver and/or elder is knowledgeable in use. Occupational therapist assists in evaluation.
  F. Relationship with caregiver:
    1. Social atmosphere—Meal sharing versus accomplishment of task.
    2. Position of care giver relative to elder—Eye contact, seating so faces are in same plane (*en face*).
    3. Pacing and choice—Care giver allows elder to choose food and determine tempo of meal; relies on elder's preference whenever known, voiced, or expressed through gestures and/or sounds.
    4. Cuing—Caregiver cues elder whenever possible with words or gestures.
    5. Self-feeding—Encouragement to self-feed with multiple methods versus assisted-feeding to minimize time.

III. EVALUATION OF EXPECTED OUTCOMES
  A. Individual
    1. Diet assessment upon admission to unit or service documented.
    2. Weight and height measured initially and weight measured at least weekly.
    3. Assessment of patient, context, and caregiver interaction after meals in which less than 50% of food offered is consumed.
    4. Diagnostic work-up, care, and treatment by interdisciplinary team, if deviations from expected nutritional norms exist.
    5. Corrective and supportive strategies reflected in plan of care.
    6. Quality of life issues emphasized in maintaining social aspects of dining.
    7. End-of-life decisions regarding nutrition respected.
  B. Health Care Provider
    1. System disruptions at mealtimes minimized.
    2. Family and paraprofessional staff informed and educated to patient's special needs to promote safe and effective meals.
    3. Maintenance of normal meals and adequate intake for the patient reflected in care plan.
    4. Competence in diet assessment; knowledge of and sensitivity to cultural norms of mealtimes reflected in care plan.
  C. Institution
    1. Documentation of nutritional status and eating and feeding behavior meets expected standard.

(continued)

TABLE 3.1 *(continued)*

2. Alterations in nutritional status, eating and feeding behaviors assessed and addressed in a timely manner.
3. Referrals to interdisciplinary team (geriatrician, advanced practice nurse (NP/CNS), dietitian, speech therapist, dentist, occupational therapist, social worker, pastoral counselor, ethicist) appropriate.
4. Nutritional, eating and/or feeding problems modified to respect individual wishes and cultural norms.

IV. FOLLOW-UP TO MONITOR CLOSELY
  A. Providers' competency to monitor nutritional status, and eating and feeding behaviors.
  B. Documentation of nutritional status, eating and feeding behaviors.
  C. Documentation of care strategies and follow-up of alterations in nutritional status, and eating and feeding behaviors.

Chapter 4

URINARY INCONTINENCE IN OLDER ADULTS

Christine Bradway, Sharon Hernly, and the
NICHE Faculty

Urinary incontinence is involuntary loss of urine sufficient to be
a problem[1]. More than 13 million adults in America are affected
by UI[2]. Adverse physiological consequences of UI commonly
encountered in acute care facilities include an increased potential
for urinary tract infection (UTI) and indwelling catheter use[3],
dermatitis, skin infections, and pressure ulcers[4]. UI that results
in functional decline can predispose older individuals to all the
complications associated with bedrest and immobility[5].

UI ETIOLOGIES

Continence requires intact lower urinary tract function, cognitive
and functional ability to recognize voiding signals and use a toilet, the motivation to maintain continence, and an environment
that facilitates the process. Micturition (urination) involves vol-
untary and reflexive control of the bladder, urethra, detrusor
muscle, and urethral sphincter. When bladder volume reaches

approximately 400 ml, stretch receptors in the bladder wall send a message to the brain, an impulse for voiding is sent back to the bladder, the detrusor muscle contracts, and the urethral sphincter relaxes to allow urination[7,8]. Normally, micturition reflexes can be inhibited voluntarily (at least for a time) until an individual desires to void or finds an appropriate place for voiding. UI occurs because of a disruption at any point during this process.

The Agency for Health Care Policy and Research (AHCPR) guideline for UI[2] identifies two types of UI: transient (acute) and established (chronic). Transient UI is characterized by the sudden onset of potentially reversible symptoms. Causes of transient UI include:

- Delirium
- Infection (e.g., untreated UTI)
- Atrophic vaginitis or urethritis
- Pharmaceuticals
- Depression or other psychological disorders that affect motivation or function
- Excessive urine production
- Restricted mobility
- Stool impaction or constipation (creating additional pressure on the bladder and causing urinary urgency and frequency)

Hospitalized elders are at risk of developing transient UI and, with shorter hospital stays, are also at risk of being discharged without resolution of the UI. However, transient UI often is preventable or at least reversible if the underlying cause is identified and treated.

Established UI has either a sudden or gradual onset and often is present before hospital admission; however, it may be discovered initially by health care providers or family caregivers during the course of an acute illness, hospitalization, or abrupt change in environment or daily routine[9]. Examples of established UI are:

Stress—defined as an involuntary loss of urine associated with activities that increase intra-abdominal pressure[2]. Symptomatically, individuals with stress UI usually present with small amounts of daytime urine loss that occur during physical activity or with increased intra-abdominal pressure(e.g., coughing, sneezing)[2]. Stress UI is more common in women, but also can be found in men after prostate surgery.

Urge—characterized by an involuntary urine loss associated with a strong desire to void (urgency)[2]. In addition to urgency , signs and symptoms of this type UI most often include frequency, nocturia, and enuresis, and UI of moderate to large amounts.

Overflow—associated with overdistention of the bladder, which may be caused by an underactive detrusor muscle or outlet obstruction[2]. Individuals with overflow UI often describe frequent, constant or postvoid dribbling; urinary retention or hesitancy; urine loss without a recognizable urge; or an uncomfortable sensation of fullness or pressure in the lower abdomen.

Functional—caused by nongenitourinary factors, such as cognitive or physical impairments, that result in an individual's inability to independently perform toileting. For example, acute physical or cognitive impairments can reduce a person's ability to recognize voiding signals, find an appropriate place to void in enough time, or be physically capable of maintaining continence.

ASSESSMENT PARAMETERS

Nurses play a key role in assessing and managing UI in hospitalized elders. Because UI is a multidisciplinary problem, collaboration with all members of the health care team is essential. Basic history and examination techniques are presented in this chapter along with a nursing standard of practice protocol outlined in Table 4.1.

History

When a patient is admitted, nursing history should include questions to determine if the individual has preexisting UI or risk factors for developing UI while hospitalized. If so, questions should focus on the incontinence characteristics: time of onset, frequency, and severity. Questions also should address possible precipitants of UI (e.g., coughing, functional decline, acute illness) and health history. Nurses also should inquire about lower urinary tract symptoms, such as nocturia, hematuria, and hesitancy, and current UI management strategies. The presence of an indwelling urinary catheter also should be documented.

TABLE 4.1   Nursing Standard of Practice Protocol: Urinary Incontinence in Older Adults Admitted to Acute Care

I.   BACKGROUND
   A. UI is the involuntary loss of urine sufficient to be a problem.
   B. UI affects approximately 13 million Americans and is prevalent in hospitalized elders,
   C. Risk factors associated with UI include immobility, impaired cognition, medications, fecal impaction, low fluid intake, environmental barriers, diabetes mellitus, and stroke.
   D. Nurses play a key role in assessing and managing UI.

II. Assessment Parameters
   A. Document the presence or absence of UI for all patients on admission.
   B. Document the presence or absence of an indwelling urinary catheter.
   C. For patients who are incontinent.
      1. Determine whether the problem is transient, established, or both.
      2. Identify and document the possible etiologies of UI.
      3. Elicit assistance with assessment and management from multidisciplinary team members.

III. Care Strategies
   A. General principles that apply to prevention and management of all forms of UI:
      1. Identify and treat causes of transient UI.
      2. Identify and continue successful prehospital management strategies for established UI.
      3. Develop an individualized plan of care using data obtained from the history and physical examination and in collaboration with other team members.
      4. Avoid medications that may contribute to UI.
      5. Avoid indwelling urinary catheters whenever possible.
      6. Monitor fluid intake and maintain an appropriate hydration schedule.
      7. Modify the environment to facilitate continence.
      8. Provide patients with usual undergarments in expectation of continence.
      9. Prevent skin breakdown by providing immediate cleansing after an incontinent episode.
      10. Use absorbent products judiciously.
   B. Strategies for specific problems:
      1. Stress UI:
         a. Teach pelvic muscle exercises (PME see Box 1).
         b. Provide toileting assistance and bladder training PRN.
         c. Consider referral to other team members if pharmacologic or surgical therapies are warranted.

(continued)

TABLE 4.1 *(continued)*

  2. Urge UI:
       a. Implement bladder training or habit training.
       b. Teach PME to be used in conjunction with a.
       c. Consider referral to other team members if pharmacologic
          therapy is warranted.
       d. Initiate referrals for patients who do not respond to the above.
  3. Overflow UI:
       a. Allow sufficient time for voiding.
       b. Instruct patients in double voiding and Credé maneuver.
       c. Consider use of external collection devices for men.
       d. Provide sterile intermittent or indwelling catheterization PRN.
       e. Initiate referrals to other team members for patients requiring
          pharmacologic or surgical intervention.
  4. Functional UI:
       a. Provide scheduled toileting or habit training.
       b. Provide adequate fluid intake.
       c. Collaborate with other team members to eliminate any
          medications adversely affecting continence.
       d. Refer for physical and occupational therapy PRN.

IV. EVALUATION OF EXPECTED OUTCOMES
   A. Patients will have fewer or no episodes of UI or complications
      associated with UI
   B. Health care providers:
      1. Will document continence status at admission and throughout
         hospital stay.
      2. Will use multidisciplinary expertise and interventions to assess
         and manage UI during hospitalization.
      3. Will include UI in discharge planning needs and
         refer PRN
   C. Institution:
      1. Will see a decrease in incidence and prevalence of acute UI.
      2. Will implement policies that require assessing and documenting
         continence status.
      3. Will provide access to AHCPR Guideline, Urinary Incontinence in
         Adults: Acute and Chronic Management[2].
      4. Will give staff administrative support and ongoing education
         regarding assessment and management of UI.

V. FOLLOW-UP TO MONITOR THE CONDITION
   A. Provide the patient and the caregiver discharge teaching regarding
      outpatient referral and management.
   B. Incorporate continuous quality improvement criteria into existing
      program.
   C. Identify areas for improvement and enlist multidisciplinary assistance
      in devising strategies for improvement.

A bladder diary or voiding record is the gold standard for obtaining objective information about the patient's voiding pattern, incontinent episodes, and UI severity. Several voiding record guides are available[1,2]; facilities may select one that best meets their needs. Advanced practice nurses or urologic and continence specialists can assist nursing staff with record interpretation and offer suggestions regarding nursing interventions based on information from the diary. A bladder diary completed for even 1 day can help identify patients with bladder dysfunction and the need for further referral.

A wide variety of medications can adversely affect continence. Nurses should document all over-the-counter and prescription medications on admission and scrutinize new medications if UI suddenly develops during the patient's hospital stay.

COMPREHENSIVE ASSESSMENT

Important components of a comprehensive examination include abdominal, genital, rectal, and the skin examinations. Inspection of male and female genitalia can be completed during bathing or as part of skin assessment. The nurse should observe the patient for signs and of perineal irritation, lesions, or discharge. In women, a Valsava maneuver (if not medically contraindicated) may identify pelvic prolapse (e.g., cystocele, rectocele, uterine prolapse) or stress UI as a result of increased intra-abdominal pressure with bearing down. Postmenopausal women are especially prone to atrophic vaginitis; significant findings include perineal inflammation, tenderness (and occasionally trauma as a result of touch), and thin, pale tissues.

Functional, environmental, and mental status assessments also are essential components of the UI evaluation in older adults. The nurse should observe the patient voiding to assess mobility, determine the need for assistive devices, and identify any obstacles that interfere with appropriate use of toilets or toilet substitutes.

CARE STRATEGIES IN ACUTE CARE

Transient causes of UI should be investigated, identified, and treated. Individuals who are admitted with a history of established UI should have their usual toileting routine and continence strategies immediately incorporated into the acute care plan as much as possible. Nurses play an essential role in initiating discharge planning and patient and caregiver teaching regarding all aspects of UI; this role also should be incorporated at admission and continuously revised as necessary.

The hospital environment should be modified to facilitate continence. Nurse call bells should be identified and placed within easy reach. If limited mobility is anticipated, nursing staff should consider using an elevated toilet seat, urinal, or bedpan. Restraints should be avoided, including side rails. Patients should be encouraged and assisted to void before leaving the unit for tests. Nurses should obtain referrals to physical and occupational therapists for ambulation aides, gait training, further assessment of activities of daily living associated with continence, and improved muscle strength. Box 1 provides helpful tips for instructing patents on performance of Pelvic Muscle Exercises (PMEs).

Decisions regarding catheterization require careful consideration of the benefits and burdens associated with their use. Indwelling urinary catheters should be avoided. Dowd and Campbell[10]

BOX 1.   Tips for Instructing Patients in Pelvic Muscle Exercises

- Explain the purpose: Pelvic muscle exercises (PMEs) or Kegel exercises strengthen the pelvic muscles and can improve stress or urge UI.
- Help patients find the correct muscle by either:
  - ◆ Verbally explaining that they should gently squeeze the rectal or vaginal muscle.
  - ◆ Manually assisting them to identify the muscle by instructing them to squeeze around your finger during a vaginal or a rectal exam.
- Instruct patients not to squeeze the stomach, buttocks, or thigh muscles (because this only increases intra-abdominal pressure) but to concentrate on isolating the pelvic muscle.
- Explain that ideally each exercise should consist of squeezing for 10 seconds and relaxing for 10 seconds. Some patients may need to start with 3 or 5 seconds and then increase as their muscles get stronger.
- Encourage patients to do 50 exercises per day but not more than 25 at once.
- Point out that patients may notice improvement in 2 to 4 weeks but not immediately. Reinforce compliance and initiate a referral for discharge follow-up with a continence specialist.

found a UTI incidence of 10% associated with their use and suggest that infections may have increased patients' hospital stays and decreased opportunities for nursing staff to identify continence as a problem or discharge need. Sterile intermittent catheterization may result in a lower incidence of infection[11] and may be a viable alternative to an indwelling catheter.

FOLLOW-UP AND SUMMARY

Although acute-care stays are generally short, UI is a significant health problem that should not be overlooked. Behavioral and supportive therapies and patient education should be initiated by nurses if the patient is cognitively, physically, and emotionally able to participate. Moreover, at discharge, hospital nurses have the responsibility of designing a plan that includes referral to a continence nurse specialist or physician for follow-up.

Continuous quality improvement (CQI) should encompass an effective urinary continence program. For example, quality indicators for UI may include appropriate documentation, prevalence of transient or established UI, use of catheters during hospitalization or on discharge, and documentation of referrals. In addition, the AHCPR guideline for UI[2] can be used clinically and throughout the facility for program development and CQI.

In summary, nurses can have a significant impact on improving the assessment and treatment of UI in hospitalized elders. Moreover, nurses can help promote changes in attitudes toward UI and provide education on individual, facilitywide, community, and national levels.

REFERENCES

[1] Urinary Continence Guideline Panel. U.S. Department of Health and Human Services, Agency for Health Care Policy and Research, Public Health Service. *Urinary Incontinence in Adults.* (Clinical Practice Guideline. AHCPR Publication No. 92–0038.) Rockville, MD: Author; March 1992.

[2] Fantl JA, Newman DK, Colling J, et al. U.S. Department of Health and Human Services, Agency for Health Care Policy and Research, Public Health Service. *Urinary Incontinence in Adults: Acute and Chronic Management.* (Clinical Practice Guideline No. 2, 1996 update. AHCPR Publication No. 96–0682.) Rockville, MD: Author; March 1996.

[3] Sier H, Ouslander J, Orzeck S. Urinary incontinence among geriatric patients in acute care hospital. *JAMA.* 1987;257:1767–71.

[4] U.S. Department of Health and Human Services, Agency for Health Care Policy and Research, Public Health Service. Pressure Ulcers in Adults: Prediction and Prevention. (Clinical Practice Guideline. No. 3 AHCPR Publication No.92–0047.) Rockville, MD: The Agency; May 1992.

[5] Harper CM, Lyles RM. Physiology and complications of bedrest. *J Am Geriatr Soc.* 1988;36:1047–54.

[6] Jirovec MM, Brink CA, Wells TJ. Nursing assessments in the inpatient geriatric population. *Nurs Clin North Am.* 1988;23:219–30.

[7] Gray M, Rayome R, Moore K. The urethral sphincter: an update. *Urol Nurs.* 1995;15:40–53.

[8] Wanich CK, Chapman EB. Long term care patient management simulations. Rowyaton, CT: Medical Age Publishing Co.;1989.

[9] Palmer MH. Urinary Continence: Assessment and Promotion. Gaithersburg, MD: Aspen; 1996.

[10] Dowd TT, Campbell JM. Urinary incontinence in the acute care setting. *Urol Nurs.* 1995;15:82–85.

[11] Terpenning MS, Allada R, Kauffaman CA. Intermittent urethral catherization in the elderly. *J Am Geriatr Soc.* 1989;37:411–6.

Chapter 5

ASSESSING COGNITIVE FUNCTION

Marquis D. Foreman, Kathleen Fletcher, Lorraine C. Mion, Lark J. Trygstad, and the NICHE Faculty

EDUCATIONAL OBJECTIVES

On completion of this chapter, the reader should be able to:
1. List five purposes of a cognitive assessment.
2. Compare and contrast three categories of cognitive decline.
3. Describe the parameters and assessment methods for a comprehensive assessment of cognitive function.
4. Compare and contrast formal and informal methods of assessing cognitive function.

Cognitive functioning encompasses the processes by which an individual perceives, registers, stores, retrieves, and uses information. In elders, cognitive functioning is particularly vulnerable to insult during an episode of illness. Given the importance and precariousness of cognitive functioning in the old, nurses' assessments of these processes are critical. The nurse's assessment of an individual's cognitive status can be instrumental in identifying the presence and monitoring the course of specific pathophysio-

Reproduced from Foreman, M., Fletcher, K, Mion, L, Trystad, L., Assessing cognitive function. *Geriatric Nursing*, 1996, *17*, 228–233. With permission from Mosby-Year Book, Inc.

logic states, for example, dementia, depression, or delirium (see Table 5.1); determining the individual's readiness to learn; establishing clinical goals; or evaluating the effectiveness of a treatment regimen. We report on a standard or practice protocol for assessing cognitive functioning (see Table 5.2).

Two caveats must be considered when cognitive function is assessed. First, when selecting an instrument to assess cognitive functioning, consider the following questions: What is the purpose of the assessment? Is the assessment for screening, monitoring, diagnosis, or more than one of these purposes? Each of these purposes requires different qualities of an instrument. Screening is conducted to determine whether an impairment is present; as a result, relatively imprecise methods are acceptable. Also, for the purposes of screening, the exact nature and cause of the impairment are considered irrelevant. Therefore screening methods will not determine whether the impairment is, for example, dementia, delirium, or depression. Conversely, methods useful for diagnostic purposes provide more precise, detailed, and comprehensive information about an individual's cognitive functioning. Diagnostic methods are used to identify the exact nature and cause of the impairment, as well as an indication of the remaining cognitive abilities of the individual. Monitoring of activities is used to determine cognitive status over time. Such measures generally are useful in documenting an individual's response to treatment.

Closely linked to the purpose of assessment is the question, "How often are the ratings to be made?" Depending on the purpose of the assessment, it may be important to assess the examinee more than once. The first assessment should occur in a well-controlled environment to provide information about the individual's maximal abilities, whereas the second should occur in a more real-world setting to provide an indication of the individual's ability to function relative to performing everyday activities. Monitoring of activities and function typically requires multiple assessments.

ASSESSMENT

Numerous instruments have been developed to evaluate an individual's cognitive functioning. These instruments range from full-

TABLE 5.1   A Comparison of the Clinical Features of Delirium, Dementia, and Depression

Clinical feature	Delirium	Dementia	Depression
Onset	Acute/subacute, depends on cause, often at	Chronic, generally insidious depends on cause	Coincides with major life changes, often abrupt
Course	Short, diurnal fluctuations in symptoms, worse at night, in darkness, and on awakening	Long, no diurnal effects, symptoms progressive yet relatively stable over time	Diurnal effects typically worse in the morning, situational fluctuations, but less than with delirium
Progression	Abrupt	Slow, but uneven	Variable, rapid or slow but even
Duration	Hours to less than 1 month, seldom longer	Month to years	At least 6 weeks, can be several months to years
Awareness	Reduced	Clear	Clear
Alertness	Fluctuates, lethargic or hypervigilant	Generally normal	Normal
Attention	Impaired, fluctuates	Generally normal	Minimal impairment, but is easily distracted
Orientation	Generally impaired, severity varies	Generally normal	Selective disorientation
Memory	Recent and immediate impaired	Recent and remote impaired	Selective or "patchy" impairment, "islands" of intact memory
Thinking	Disorganized, fragmented, incoherent speech, either slow or accelerated	Difficulty with abstraction, thoughts impoverished, judgment impaired, words difficult to find	Intact but with themes of hopelessness, or self-deprecation
Perception	Distorted, illusions, delusions, and hallucinations, difficulty distinguishing between reality and misperceptions	Misperceptions usually absent	Intact, delusions and hallucinations absent except in severe cases

(continued)

TABLE 5.1 A Comparison of the Clinical Features of Delirium, Dementia, and Depression

Clinical feature	Delirium	Dementia	Depression
Psychomotor behavior	Variable, hypokinetic, and mixed	Normal, may have apraxis	Variable, psychomotor retardation or agitation
Sleep/wake cycle	Disturbed, cycle reversed	Fragmented	Disturbed, usually early morning awakening
Associated	Variable affective changes, symptoms of autonomic hyperarousal exaggeration of personality type, associated with acute physical illness	Affect tends to be superficial, inappropriate and labile, attempts to conceal deficits in intellect, personality changes, aphasia, agnosia may be present, lacks insight	Affect depressed, dysphoric mood, exaggerated and detailed complaints, preoccupied with personal thoughts, insight present, verbal elaboration
Assessment	Distracted from task, numerous errors	Failings highlighted by family frequent "near miss" answers, struggles with test, great effort to find an appropriate reply, frequent requests for feedback on performance	Failings highlighted by individual, frequently answers, "don't know," little effort, frequently gives up, indifferent toward test, does not care or attempt to find answer

scale batteries that require an exquisitely skilled examiner and place intense demand on the examinee, to instruments that can be used at the bedside and place little demand on the examiner and examinee. Additionally, some of these instruments are constructed to assess a single process (e.g., attention) in great detail versus others that assess the spectrum of cognitive processes, including affect and function.

Each approach has its advantages and disadvantages. An advantage of assessing only a single cognitive process is that it minimizes the demands on the examiner and examinee; however, focusing the assessment on a single process, such as orientation, may overlook an important deficit in another, such as judgment.

TABLE 5.2   Overview of Cognitive Assessment

I. Concepts and categories
    A. Definition: Cognitive function: the processes by which an individual
       perceives, registers, retrieves, and uses information.
    B. Categories of cognitive change/decline.
       1. The dementias (e.g., Alzheimer's, vascular) are chronic,
          progressive, insidious, and permanent states of cognitive
          impairment.
       2. Delirium/acute confusion: An acute and sudden impairment of
          cognition that is considered temporary; generally an identifiable,
          biophysical cause.
       3. Impairment in thought processes

II. ASSESSMENT
    A. Methods of assessment
       1. Formal--Cognitive testing using standardized instruments.
          a. Advantages: Standardized; enables comparison across
             individuals and nurses
          b. Disadvantages: Individual performance influenced by pain,
             education, fatigue, cultural background, and perceptual and
             physical abilities.
       2. Informal--through structured observations of nurse-individual
          interactions.
          a. Advantages: May have greater meaning about individual's
             actual cognitive ability/performance.
          b. Disadvantages: Difficult to make judgments regarding change
             in individual condition; variability in interpretation.
    B. Other considerations for assessment.
       1. Characteristics of the environment for assessment.
          a. Physical environment.
             i.   Comfortable ambient temperature.
             ii. Adequate lighting but not glaring.
             iii. Free of distractions, e.g., should be conducted in the
                  absence of others and other activities.
             iv. Position self to maximize individuals' sensory abilities.
          b. Interpersonal environment.
             i.   Use individual's self-paced rate for assessment.
             ii. Emotionally nonthreatening.
       2. Timing considerations.
          a. Timing should reflect the actual cognitive abilities of the
             individual and not extraneous factors.
          b. Times of the day to generally avoid.
             i.   Immediately on awakening from sleep, wait at least 30
                  minutes-immediately before or after meals.

(continued)

TABLE 5.2   *(continued)*

ii. Immediately before or after medical diagnostic or
therapeutic procedures.
iii. When patient has pain or discomfort.
C. PARAMETERS OF ASSESSMENT
  1. Alertness/level of consciousness: The most rudimentary cognitive
function and level of arousal or responsiveness to stimuli
determined by interaction with individual and determination of
level made on the basis of the individual's best eye, verbal, and
motor response to stimuli.
   a. Alertness-Able to interact in meaningful way with the examiner.
   b. Lethargy or somnolence-Not fully alert; individual tends to
drift to sleep when not stimulated, diminished spontaneous
physical movement, loses train of thought, ideas wander.
   c. Obtundation-Transitional stage between lethargy and stupor;
difficult to arouse, meaningful testing futile, requires constant
stimulation to elicit response.
   d. Stupor or semicoma-Individual mumbles/groans in response to
persistent and vigorous physical stimulation.
   e. Coma-Completely unable to be aroused, no behavioral
response to stimuli.
  2. Attention: Ability to attend/concentrate on stimuli: can follow
through with direction, especially a three-stage command; is easily
distracted.
  3. Memory: Ability to register, retain, and recall information both
new and old; does individual remember your name? Is individual
able to learn and remember new information?
  4. Orientation to time, place, and person.
  5. Thinking: Ability to organize and communicate ideas; thoughts
should be organized, coherent, and appropriate.
  6. Perception: Presence/absence of illusions, delusions, or visual or
auditory hallucinations.
  7. Psychomotor behavior: Ability to comprehend and perform simple
motor skills. Relative to execution ability, ask the individual to
perform certain ADLs/IADLs, or to perform a three-step
command and to copy a figure.
  8. Insight: Ability to understand oneself and the situation in which
one finds oneself.
  9. Judgement: Ability to evaluate a situation (real or hypothetical)
and determine an appropriate action.

III. OUTCOMES OF ASSESSMENT
   A. Individual.
      1. Detection of deviations will be prompt and early, with appropriate
care and treatment instituted in a timely manner.

(continued)

TABLE 5.2 *(continued)*

    2. Plans of care will appropriately address corrective and supportive cognitive function.

  B. Health care provider.

    1. Assessment and documentation of cognitive function.

    2. Appropriate strategies to address any deviation in cognitive function.

    3. Competence in cognitive assessment.

    4. Evidence of ability to differentiate among the different types of cognitive change/decline.

  C. Institution.

    1. Documentation of cognitive function will increase.

    2. Referral to appropriate advanced practitioners (e.g., geriatrician, geriatric/gerontological or psychiatric clinical nurse specialist or nurse practitioner, or consultation-liaison service) will increase.

ADL, Activities of daily living: IADL, instrumental activities of daily living.
Adapted from Abraham et al.[3], Foreman and Grabowski[4], Mandell et al.[5], Smith et al.[6], Strub and Black[7], Tombaugh and McIntyre[8], Dellasega[9], and Milisen et al.[10].

Conversely, an assessment of all cognitive processes provides a global indication of the individual's cognitive abilities, but it is time-consuming, places intensive demands on the examinee, and may be less sensitive to some aspects of cognition. An extensive review of these instruments is reported elsewhere[1].

SELECTING AN INSTRUMENT

What level of impairment is to be assessed? It is important to select an instrument that is adequate for the level of impairment. An instrument may be highly sensitive to a part of the spectrum of impairment; for example, it may be useful for mild to moderate impairment and insensitive to differences at the severe range. For example, many instruments will rate an individual with dementia as having severe cognitive impairment, but will be unable to differentiate an individual who is totally dependent for care from an individual who can still walk and feed himself or herself.

For what specific subpopulation is the instrument designed? The answer to this question will assist in determining the general content and level of functioning that is assessed by the instrument. Examples of subpopulations are individuals who are educationally disadvantaged, who speak English as a second language, or who have various physical handicaps. An instrument for cognitive assessment may also be selected on the basis of abilities or handicaps of the examinee. Lezak[2] provides an excellent discussion of features to be considered when selecting an instrument for use with individuals with sensory-motor handicaps or those with severe brain damage. Additional characteristics of the examinee to consider are age, educational level, race, and socioeconomic level.

Should subjective (individual self-reports) and objective (observations or testing by the nurse or some other) ratings be distinguished? Again, the answer to this question will be influenced by many of the previous questions. Subjective and objective evidence is often critical to an accurate diagnosis.

In the use of an instrument, the comfort and privacy of both the examiner and examinee should be considered. The room should be well lit and set at a comfortable ambient temperature, so that neither the examiner nor the examinee is distracted from the cognitive task. Lighting must be balanced to be sufficient for the examinee to see the examination materials adequately, although not being so bright as to create glare. Laminated materials create glare. Positioning is important relative to fighting and glare. Also, the assessment environment should be free from distractions that can result from extraneous noise, assessment materials should not be scattered about, nor should brightly colored or patterned clothing and flashy jewelry be worn by the examiner[2].

Performing the assessment in the presence of others should be avoided when possible, because the other individual can be distracting. If the other is a significant intimate relative, additional problems arise. For example, when the examinee fails to respond or responds in error, the significant other has been known to provide the answer, or to say, "Now, you know the answer to that" or "Now, you know that's wrong." In most instances, the presence of another only serves to heighten anxiety.

The assessment environment should be emotionally nonthreatening. For example, older adults are especially sensitive to any insinuation that they may have some "memory problem." Therefore the dilemma for the examiner is to stress the importance of the assessment while taking care not to increase the examinee's anxiety by asking the older about memory problems; explaining that these often occur with various diseases is useful. It is important to create an environment in which the examinee is motivated to perform and to perform well, while not being overly anxious and thereby perform poorly. It is counterproductive to describe the assessment as consisting of "simple," "silly," or "stupid" questions. Anxiety is heightened after a series of failures on assessment. Lezak[2] suggests altering the order of the presentation of items so that the examinee can have some experience with success.

Various characteristics of the examiner and examinee also should be considered. Many of the instruments to assess cognitive functioning can be perceived by the examinee as intrusive, intimidating, fatiguing, and offensive–characteristics that can seriously and negatively affect performance. Consequently, Lezak[2] recommends a 15–to 20–minute period to establish rapport with the examinee. This period also allows a determination of the examinee's capacity for tolerating the assessment. For example, this period can be used to determine special problems that could influence testing or its interpretation (e.g., sensory decrements). With elderly individuals who may have some decrements in sensory abilities, the examiner can improve the examinee's ability to perform through simple methods. For example, if the examinee has any degree of hearing impairment, taking a position across from the examiner or a little to the side may enhance the examinee's hearing. In this position, the examinee can readily use the examiner's nonverbal communication, as well as read the examiner's lips. Sitting a little to the side of the ear with the better auditory function of the examinee also improves the examinee's hearing.

Cognitive assessment can be fatiguing to both the examiner and examinee. Thus examiners are cautioned to be alert for fatigue, because not all examinees will inform the examiner they are becoming fatigued. Lezak[2] recommends observing for physical evidence of being tired-slurring of speech, motor slowing, and restlessness. When the examinee is fatigued, temporarily terminating the assessment should be considered. Many of the assessment instruments can be administered in sections; however, if the assessment must be terminated in the middle of a section, it would be wise to repeat the entire section.

Clearly, certain times of the day are inappropriate for obtaining reliable and valid assessments of cognitive functioning. Times of the day that generally should be avoided are immediately on awakening from sleep, immediately before and after meals, immediately before and after medical diagnostic and therapeutic procedures, or when the examinee has discomfort or pain. The timing of the assessment should be selected to best reflect the true abilities of the individual and not extraneous factors.

Interpretation of the results of cognitive assessment is not simple and should consist of more than just the score obtained on testing. The following must be considered when the results of the cognitive assessment are interpreted: the nature and pattern of the examinee's responses to testing, the examinee's behavior during testing, the context of the assessment, the examinee's health history, physical examination results, and results of various laboratory and other tests, educational level, occupation, family history, current living situation, and level of social functioning, and presence of sensory or motor deficits.

The nature and pattern of the responses to testing can also provide valuable information about an individual's cognitive status. Noting the examinee's verbatim responses on testing is often valuable in differential diagnosis.

Anecdotal notes of the context of testing, the testing environment, and the appearance of the examinee during testing also are important for better understanding the performance on testing. Supplementary information from the examinee's health history, physical examination result, and laboratory and other test results can provide valuable insight into the individual's performance on testing.

Clearly, the determination of an individual's cognitive status is important in the process and outcomes of illness and its treatment. Being competent in the assessment of cognitive functioning requires the following: (1) knowledge and skill as they relate to the performance of a cognitive assessment, (2) sensitivity to the issues that can negatively bias the results of this assessment, (3) accurate and comprehensive documentation of the assessment, and (4) the incorporation of the results of the assessment in the development of the individual's plan of care.

REFERENCES

[1]   Foreman MD. Measuring cognitive status. In: Frank-Strombborg M, Olsen S, Eds. *Instruments for Clinical Research in Health Care,* 2nd ed. Wilsonville, OR: Jones and Barlett; 1997.

[2]   Lezak MD. *Neuropsychological Assessment,* 3rd ed. New York: Oxford University Press; 1995.

[3]   Abraham IL, Manning CA, Snustad DG, Brashear HR, Newman MC, Wofford AB. Cognitive screening of nursing home residents: Factor structures of the Mini-Mental State Examination. *J Am Geriatr Soc.* 1994;42:750–756.

[4]   Foreman MD, Grabowski R. Diagnostic dilemma: Cognitive impairment in the elderly. *J Gerontol Nurs.* 1992;18(9):5–12.

[5]   Mandell AM, Knoefel JE, Albert ML. Mental status examination in the elderly. In: Albert ML, Knoefel JE. *Clinical Neurology of Aging,* 2nd ed. New York: Oxford University Press; 1994:277–313.

[6]   Smith MJ, Breitbart WS, Platt MM. A critique of instruments and methods to detect, diagnose, and rate delirium. *J Pain Symptom Manage.* 1995;10:35–77.

[7]   Strub RL, Black FW. *The Mental Status Examination in Neurology,* 2nd ed. Philadelphia: Davis, 1985.

[8]   Tombaugh TN, McIntyre NJ. The Mini-Mental State Examination: A Comprehensive Review. *J Am Geriatr Soc.* 1992;40:922–35.

[9]   Dellaseca C. Assessment of Cognition in the Elderly. Pieces of a Complex Puzzle. *Nurs Clin North Am.* 1998;33(3):395–405.

[10] Milisen K, Foreman MD, Godderis J, Abraham IL, & Broos PLO. Delirium in the hospitalized elderly. Nursing assessment and management. *Nurs Clin North Am.* 1998;33(3):417–439.

Chapter 6

ACUTE CONFUSION/DELIRIUM: STRATEGIES FOR ASSESSING AND TREATING

Marquis D. Foreman, Lorraine C. Mion,
Lark J. Trygstad, Kathleen Fletcher, and the
NICHE Faculty

EDUCATIONAL OBJECTIVES

On completion of this chapter, the reader should be able to:
1. List the four(4) most common causes of delirium/acute confusion.
2. Describe two characteristics of the etiologic basis of delirium/acute confusion.
3. Identify patients at risk for an episode of delirium/acute confusion
4. Develop a plan of care for a delirious patient.

STANDARD OF PRACTICE PROTOCOL: ACUTE CONFUSION/DELIRIUM

Acute confusion, also known as delirium, is a prevalent syndrome, and one of the major contributors to poor outcomes of health care

and institutionalization of elders. It is characterized by a disturbance of consciousness with reduced ability to focus, sustain, or
shift attention; a change in cognition; or the development of a
perceptual disturbance, which develops over a short period of
time and tends to fluctuate during the course of the day[1]. These
disturbances may be manifested by hypervigilance or inattentive-
ness; disorientation; memory impairment; and illusions, hallucinations, or misperceptions of stimuli. These symptoms are reflected
in behavior that appears inappropriate or unusual for the individual. The severity of these symptoms varies during the day, typically being worse in the evening or when the patient is fatigued[2].

The onset generally occurs shortly after admission to the hospital, usually between the second and third days; few cases develop
after the sixth day of hospitalization[2]. The duration of acute
confusion is highly variable and depends in part on how quickly
it and its causes are identified, and how promptly and accurately
treatment is initiated[3]. On average, however, acute confusion
lasts less than 5 days; cases of delirium lasting longer than 7 days
are rare[2,3].

Confused patients more frequently experience adverse reactions
to therapeutic doses of medications, fall, develop pressure ulcers,
and develop infections. Because of their inability to think clearly,
acutely confused patients are unable to care for themselves, and
frequently exhibit unsafe behaviors, thus, they require greater
nursing surveillance[4], and for which they are more frequently
physically restrained[5]. Also, the length of hospitalization is protracted for these patients, frequently beyond that for which hospitals are compensated[6,7].

Despite variability in the etiologic basis of acute confusion, there
is agreement[2] about the most common causes of acute confusion: (1) medication, especially those drugs with anticholinergic
properties, or those that have potent central nervous system effects, for example, diphenhydramine (Benadryl); (2) infection,
particularly urinary tract and respiratory infections; (3) dehydration and electrolyte imbalance, especially hypo-or hypernatremia,
and hypo-or hyperkalemia; and (4) metabolic disturbances such
as azotemia, pH alterations, and nutritional deficiencies.

To summarize, the etiologic basis of acute confusion is: (1)
multifactorial, comprising physiologic, psychologic, sociologic, and

environmental elements; and, (2) dynamic meaning that the causes of acute confusion vary across time and specific patient populations. Together these characteristics of the etiologic basis of acute confusion make the diagnosis of specific causes complex and elusive-a diagnostic dilemma that challenges even the most skillful clinicians[see Box 1 for details][8].

NURSING STRATEGIES FOR ACUTE CONFUSION

Once it has been determined that the patient is either at risk for becoming acutely confused or is already acutely confused, the question remains, "What can be done to either prevent or treat the acute confusion?" The following principles have been set forth to guide in the effective prevention and treatment of acute confusion. The first principle is to prevent, eliminate, or minimize the etiologic agent(s). These strategies include administering medications judiciously, preventing infection, maintaining fluid volume, and promoting electrolyte balance. The second principle is to provide a therapeutic environment and general supportive nursing care [see Box 2, pp. 69–75][8].

SUMMARY AND CONCLUSIONS

Acute confusion is a common occurrence in many hospitalized elders. Thus, it is important to promptly identify those patients at risk for an acute confusion or those presently confused. To do so, nursing assessments must become routine and systematic. In addition, the assessment of cognition should be comprehensive. A standard of practice protocol provides concise information to guide nursing care of individuals at risk of or experiencing acute confusion. This clinical practice protocol covers the background issues, risk factors, clinical assessment, care strategies and evaluation of expected outcomes necessary to optimally assess and treat acute confusion/delirium. Additional recent references are included at

Box 1. Assessing for Acute Confusion/Delirium		
Feature	Assessment parameters	Findings if acute confusion
Alertness	Level of consciousness: observation of behavior -alert (normal) -vigilant (hyperalert) -lethargic (drowsy but easily aroused) -stupor (difficult to arouse) -coma (unarousable)	Fluctuates from stuporous to hypervigilant
Attention	Ability to attend/concentrate: through naturally occurring conversation, observation of behavior, or formal testing using: -Digit span, forward and backward -Vigilance "A" test -Serial subtraction -Spelling backwards	Inattentive, easily distractible, and may have difficulty shifting attention from one focus to another; has difficulty keeping track of
Orientation	Questioning about orientation to person, place, and time: through naturally occurring observation or formal testing.	Disoriented to time and place; should not be disoriented to person.
Memory	Questioning about recent and remote events. Day-to-day observation	Inability to recall events of hospitalization and illness; unable to remember instructions; forgetful of names, events, activities, current news, etc.
Thinking	Naturally occurring conversation	disorganized thinking; rambling, irrelevant, incoherent conversation; unclear or illogical flow of ideas; or unpredictable switching from topic to topic; difficulty in expressing needs and concerns; speech may be garbled.
Perception	Recognition of objects and persons.	Perceptual disturbances, such as illusions and hallucinations, and

(continued)

Box 1. *(continued)*		
Feature	Assessment parameters	Findings if acute confusion
Psychomotor behavior	Observation of behavior -Hypo- or hyperkinetic -Unusual or inappropriate Day-to-day interaction	misperceptions such as calling a stranger by a relative's name Variable, from sluggish and moving very slowly to restlessness and agitation. Behavior that is considered unusual for that individual or inappropriate for the situation.

Adapted from Foreman and Zane[8].

the end of this chapter to enable the clinician to find additional resources regarding this topic[4,9-24].

REFERENCES

[1] American Psychiatric Association. *Diagnostic and statistical manual of mental disorders* (4th ed.). Washington, DC: Author; 1994.

[2] Foreman, MD. Acute confusion in the elderly. *Ann Rev Nurs Res.* 1993;11:3–30.

[3] Rudberg MA., Pompei P, Foreman MD, Ross RE, Cassel CK. The natural history of delirium in older hospitalized patients: A syndrome of heterogeneity. *Age Ageing.* 1997;26:169–174.

[4] Williams MA, Ward SE, Campbell EB. Confusion: Testing versus observation. *J Gerontol Nurs.* 1988;14(1):25–30.

[5] Sullivan-Marx E. Delirium and physical restraint in the hospitalized elderly. *Image.* 1994;26:295–300.

[6] Francis J, Hilko E, Kapoor N. Delirium and prospective payment: The economic impact of confusion [abstract]. *J Am Geriatr Soc.* 1994;41(Suppl):SA9.

[7] Pompei P, Foreman MD, Rudberg MA, Inouye SK, Braund V, Cassel CK. Delirium in hospitalized older persons: Outcomes and predictors. *J Am Geriatri Soc.* 1994;42:809–815.

[8]   Foreman MD, Zane D. Nursing strategies for acute confusion in hospitalized elderly patients. *Am J Nurs.* 1996;96(4):44–51.

[9]   Foreman MD, Fletcher K, Mion LC, Simon L, the NICHE Faculty. Assessing cognitive function. *Geriatr Nurs.* 1996;17(5):228–233.

[10] Cole MG, Primeau F, McCusker J. Effectiveness of interventions to prevent delirium in hospitalized patients: A systematic review. *Canad Med Assoc J.* 1996;155:1263–1268.

[11] Cole MG, Primeau FJ, Bailey RF, Bonnycastel MJ, Masciarelli F, Engelsmann F, Pepin MJ, Ducic D. Systematic intervention for elderly inpatients with delirium: A randomized trial. *Canad Med Assoc J.* 1994;151:965–970.

[12] Cronin-Stubbs D. (1996). Delirium intervention research in acute care settings. *Ann Rev Nurs Res.* 1996;14:57–71.

[13] Matthiesen V, Sivertsen L, Foreman MD, Cronin-Stubbs D. Acute confusion: Nursing intervention in older patients. *Ortho Nurs.* 1994;13(2):21–29.

[14] Morency CR. Mental status change in the elderly: Recognizing and treating delirium. *J Prof Nurs.* 1990;6:356–365.

[15] Nagley SJ, Dever A. What we know about treating confusion. *Appl Nurs Res.* 1988;1:80–83.

[16] Neelon VJ. Postoperative delirium. *CC Nurs Clin N Am.* 1990;2:579–587.

[17] Neelon VJ, Champagne MT. Managing cognitive impairment: The current basis for practice. In Funk SG, Tournquist EM, Champagne MT, Wiese RA (Eds.), *Key aspects of elder care: Managing falls, incontinence, and cognitive impairment.* New York: Springer; 1992, 239–250.

[18] Ribby KJ, Cox KR. Development, implementation, and evaluation of a confusion protocol. *Clin Nurs Spec.* 1996;10:241–247.

[19] Walker MK, Foreman MD, the NICHE Faculty. Ensuring medication safety for older adults. New York: Springer; 1999, pp. 000–000.

[20] Wanich CK, Sullivan-Marx EM, Gottlieb GL, Johnson JC. Functional status outcomes of a nursing intervention in hospitalized elderly. *Image.* 1992;24:201–207.

[21] Williams MA. The physical environment and patient care. *Ann Rev Nurs Res.* 1988;7:61–84.

[22] Williams MA, Campbell EB, Raynor WW Jr, Mlynarczyk SM, Ward SE. Reducing acute confusional states in elderly patients with hip fractures. *Res Nurs Health.* 1985;8:329–337.

[23] Wolanin MO, Phillips LRF. *Confusion: Prevention and care.* St. Louis: Mosby; 1981.

[24] Yeaw EMJ, Abbate JH. Identification of confusion among the elderly in an acute care setting. *Clin Nurs Spec.* 1993;7:192–197.

Box 2. Nursing Strategies for Acute Confusion		
Etiologic agent	Physical findings	Nursing actions

Medications
 	
Special attention
Anticholinergic
  preparations
• thioridazine
• amitriptypine
• neuroleptics
• tricyclic
  antidepressants
• atropine
• theophylline
• diphenhydramine
Histamine-2
  blocking agents
• cimetidine
• ranitidine
Analgesics
• meperidine
• non-steroidal
  anti-inflammatory
  agents
Sedative-hypnotics
• halcion
• benzodiazepines
Cardiovascular drugs
• nifedipine
• quinidine
	variable, depending on
	the specific medication
	drug–drug interactions
	and the person's
	underlying health
	problems and health
	status.
		Monitor the effects
		(intended and adverse) of
		medications. Be especially
		vigilant for drug
		interactions. With the
		onset of any new
		symptom, first consider
		it as an adverse reaction
		to a medication.
		
		Encourage and administer
		only those medications
		indicated by the patient's
		status, thereby keeping
		medication to a minimum.
		
		Relieve pain through
		adequate and appropriate
		administration of analgesia
		and alternative therapies.
		
		Refer to/notify appropriate
		advanced practice nurse or
		house officer
		
		Document actions and
		patient response in
		hospital record

Infection
 	
Most common:
  Urinary tract
  Respiratory
 	
Most overlooked:
  Mouth
  Feet
	Urinary:
	-Dysuria is frequently
	  absent
	-Frequency
	-Urgency
	-Nocturia
	-Incontinence
	-Anorexia
	-Cultures may be
	  negative
	-Protein and/or blood
	  dipstick
		Determine source and site
		of infection
		
		Provide adequate fluids,
		2000 ml per day, unless
		otherwise contraindicated
		
		Apply cooling techniques
		as needed, and indicated,
		e.g., remove covers or use
		cooling mattress/blanket
		(continued)

	Box 2. *(continued)*	
Etiologic agent	Physical findings	Nursing actions
	Respiratory: -Cough may be dry, productive, or absent -Slight cyanosis -Anorexia -Nausea -Vomiting -Tachycardia -Chills, fever, and elevated WBC may not be present -Cultures may be negative -Breath sounds: wheezes, crackles, or gurgles possible -Change in patient's functional level often seen as first sign	Monitor for flushed hot skin, tachycardia, seizures changes in body temperature, and breath sounds q 2 h or as indicated by status of the patient Monitor intake and output For resp., provide humidified air, cough and deep breath PRN, provide frequent oral hygiene; CPT to mobilize secretions Refer to/notify appropriate advanced practice nurse or house officer
Dehydration	Hypotension with orthostatic changes evident Tachycardia Hyperthermia Weakness Nausea Anorexia Oliguria Dry mucous membranes & skin Poor skin turgor Increased thirst	Determine source of dehydration, e.g., decreased fluid intake or increased fluid output Check medications as a cause for increased loss of fluids, e.g., diuretics Check the person's ability to swallow or for mechanical problems preventing fluid intake Refer to/notify appropriate advanced practice nurse or house officer

(continued)

Box 2. *(continued)*		
Etiologic agent	Physical findings	Nursing actions
		Prepare for fluid replace and additional diagnostic and therapeutic actions
		Continue surveillance of patient q 2–6 hours as indicated by patient status
		Document actions and patient response in hospital record
Hypokalemia (< 3.5 mEq/L)	Hypotension Tachycardia Weakness Apathy Constipation Fatigue Lethargy Tachyarrhythmias Low serum potassium	Determine source of hypokalemia, e.g., inadequate intake of potassium, rich foods, excessive loss due to the effects of medications (non-potassium sparing diuretics)
		Refer to/notify appropriate advanced practice nurse or house officer
		Document actions and patient response in hospital record
Hypernatremia (> 146 mEq/L)	Weight loss Orthostatic hypotension Increased thirst Poor skin turgor, dry mucous membranes Oliguria Lethargy Hyperthermia Elevated HCT, BUN, creatinine, and serum osmolarity	Determine source of hypenatremia, e.g., increased water loss (fever, infection, vomiting, diarrhea), decreased water intake (physical or cognitive limitations), or increased sodium intake
		Prepare for electrolyte and possibly fluid replacement

(continued)

Box 2. *(continued)*		
Etiologic agent	Physical findings	Nursing actions
		Restrict activity to maintain energy balance
		Continue to monitor parameters q 2 h or as indicated by status of patient
		Refer to/notify appropriate advanced practice nurse or house officer
		Document actions and patient response in hospital record
Hyponatremia (< 136 mEq/L)	Hypotension Tachycardia Hyperthermia Nausea Malaise Lethargy Somnolence	Determine source of hyponatremia, e.g., inadequate intake of sodium, renal disease, fluid restriction, SIADH, overdiuresis
	Poor skin turgor Increased thirst Decreased serum sodium and osmolality	Prepare for electrolyte and possibly fluid replacement
	Elevated BUN, Hct, and serum proteins	Restrict activity to maintain energy balance
		Continue to monitor parameters q 2 h or as indicated by status of patient
		Refer to/notify appropriate advanced practice nurse or house officer
		Document actions and patient response in hospital record
		(continued)

Box 2. *(continued)*		
Etiologic agent	Physical findings	Nursing actions
Hypoxia	Hypertension Tachycardia Tachypnea Cyanosis (peripheral & central) Agitation Increased depth of respirations Decreased pO_2 Accessory muscle use Paradoxical breathing pattern	Determine source of hypoxia, e.g., infection, COPD, PE, bronchospasm Position patient to facilitate air exchange, e.g., high Fowler's as tolerated by patient Restrict/pace activity to reduce additional oxygen requirements Monitor blood gas results or that of pulse oximetry Refer to/notify appropriate advanced practice nurse or house officer Continue to monitor parameters q 2 h or as indicated by status of patient Prepare for oxygen administration Document actions and patient response in hospital record
Environmental challenge	Variable, depending on whether the environmental challenge presents as sensory overload or sensory deprivation	Provide explanations of nursing care and all diagnostic and therapeutic activities Position patient in a semi-Fowler's position as tolerated

(continued)

Box 2. *(continued)*		
Etiologic agent	Physical findings	Nursing actions
		Minimize abrupt relocations, otherwise, prepare patient by providing explanations of the event, send a health care provider or family member to accompany patient
		Provide orienting stimuli: clock, watch, calendar, radio, television, newspapers, personal items from home
		Encourage social interaction with friends and family
		Maintain continuity of care
		Limit the number of staff involved in the care of the patient
		Assure adequate sleep (avoid disruptions)
		Remove meaningless and unnecessary stimuli, e.g., unneeded equipment and supplies, television off when not desired, etc.
		Alternate periods of rest and activity
		Communicate clearly and simply
		Refer to/notify appropriate advanced practice nurse or house officer
		(continued)

Box 2. *(continued)*		
Etiologic agent	Physical findings	Nursing actions
		Document actions and patient's response in hospital record
Sensory Impairment	Misperceptions of visual and auditory stimuli, e.g., hallucinations, illusions, mistaking objects and persons for others	Assist patient in accurately interpreting environmental stimuli by having patient use appropriate sensory aids; also, ensure that aids are in proper working
	Diminished hearing acuity	Eliminate sources of distraction (auditory and visual)
	Diminished visual acuity	Speak clearly and slowly, do not shout, repeat key phrases as necessary
		Speak directly into the patient's "best" ear
		Face the patient when speaking so that lip reading can be used to facilitate understanding as necessary
		With written materials, use large print with lighter colored objects on darker backgrounds, place them directly in front of the patient, and use indirect lighting to reduce/eliminate glare
		Refer to/notify appropriate advanced practice nurse or house officer
		Document actions and patient's response in hospital record

Adapted from Foreman and Zane (1996).

Chapter 7

PREVENTING FALLS IN ACUTE CARE

Barbara Corrigan, Karen Allen, Janet Moore, Patricia Samra, Cheryl Stetler, Joyce Thielen, and the NICHE Faculty

EDUCATIONAL OBJECTIVES:

On completion of this chapter the reader should be able to:
1. Describe the impact of a fall as an event in the life of an older person.
2. Identify evidence-based risk factors associated with potential for patient falls.
3. Plan risk-related interventions for fall prevention.
4. Explain the role of data collection and analysis in a fall-prevention program.

BACKGROUND

As the United States population ages, there is an increase in the proportion of elderly patients receiving care in hospitals. The shift to an older, more vulnerable population is accompanied by a higher risk for falls and related injuries. A fall may result in prolonged bedrest, soft-tissue changes, pneumonia, fractures, depression, discomfort, dependency, and immobility. Even when falls do not result in physical injury, 25% of those who fall will subsequently limit their normal activities and become socially isolated because of the fear of falling again[1]. Baraff[2] explains, "A fall may be viewed as a sentinel event in the life of an older person, potentially marking the beginning of a serious decline in function" (p. 480).

Although age alone is not a risk factor, well over 50% of all falls in the hospital occur in persons over 65 years of age. There are a number of age-related changes that may contribute to falls and related injuries. These aging changes include altered visual acuity, decreased reaction time, decreased bladder capacity and contractility, demineralization of bone, decreased balance and muscle strength, and risk for orthostatic hypotension.

Falls are the second leading cause of death from trauma in the United States. For persons 65 years of age and over, falls are responsible for one-third of deaths due to injury. The number of deaths associated with falls may be grossly underestimated, as physicians do not always accurately record falls as a cause of death on the death certificate[3]. Hip fractures are a serious consequence of falls in the elderly population. More than 90% of such fractures occur in persons over 70 years of age. A study by Marottoli, et al.[4] found that 20% of those suffering a hip fracture died within 6 months, and all of the survivors had a substantial decline in physical function at 6 weeks and at 6 months.

Patient falls are the single largest category of incidents in acute care hospitals[5]. Maciorowski et al.[6] stated that 70% to 80% of all incident reports in an acute care setting were related to patient falls, and 20% to 30% of falls resulted in injury. Falls are the most common reason that nurses are sued for negligence[7]. Most fall litigation never reaches the courtroom; however, the average non-injury award is $10,000 to $15,000[7].

Nurses are in a key position to prevent falls in acute care hospitals. This chapter describes a Fall Prevention Program implemented at Baystate Medical Center, Springfield, MA which utilizes the research-based Hendrich Fall Risk Assessment Tool[8] as a foundation for implementation. A nursing standard of practice protocol is included.

Definition of a Fall

A vast body of literature has evolved on the subject of falls, yet not all authors define "fall" or describe the circumstances commonly surrounding a fall. A number of authors have noted that a standard definition of a fall is lacking[9]. From those descriptive articles or studies where a fall has been defined, the following composite definition has been developed: an unintentional or unplanned event in which the person comes to rest on the ground or floor, with or without subsequent injury[8,10–12].

For consistent data collection and analysis it is imperative that each institution develop an operational definition of a fall[13–14]. The definition of a fall used in this protocol is

> An event which results in the patient, or any part of the patient's body coming to rest inadvertently on the floor or other surface lower than the patient, including an event where a patient is found on the floor unable to account for his/her situation.

There is an inconsistency that exists in the literature regarding inclusion of a "near fall": that is, those individuals who would have fallen if not for the assistance of staff. The definition in this protocol excludes those patients who are intentionally eased to the floor by staff members and do not sustain injury. (See Box 1 for definition of a fall.)

Categories of Fall Risk Factors

Prediction of falls has been associated largely with the identification of a set of existing risk factors[8,10,15–20]. Some authors have identified an extensive, generic list of risk factors, whereas others separate them into categories. To facilitate clarification and identification of risk factors, this protocol subdivides risk factors into 3 categories: extrinsic, intrinsic/anticipated physiological, and intrinsic/unanticipated physiological[7,8,20,21]. Categories of risk factors are described in Table 7.1.

BOX 1.   Nursing Standard Of Practice Protocol: Prevention of Falls

---

I.   Goal: Reduce Patient Falls and Fall Related Injuries
   Purpose: The following nursing care protocol is designed to assist the
   professional nurse to:
   A. utilize an evidenced based method of assessing for fall.
   B. provide an objective basis for planning nursing interventions for
       fall prevention.
II. DEFINITION OF A FALL:
   A fall is defined as an event which results in the patient or any part of
   the patient's body coming to rest inadvertently on the floor, or other
   surface lower than the patient.
   A. Included in this definition are patients found lying on the floor
       unable to account for their situation.
   B. Excluded are patients who are intentionally eased to the floor by
       staff members and do not sustain an injury.
III. CATEGORIES OF FALL RISK
   A. Extrinsic: External or environmental risk factors.
   B. Intrinsic/anticipated physiological: patient characteristics or
       diagnoses that can be measured to predict a patient's likelihood to
       fall.
   C. Intrinsic/unanticipated physiological falls: unforeseeable if no
       previous history is present and no risk factors are identified from
       physical/functional assessment.
IV. ASSESSMENT OF FALL RISK:
   A. Assess all patients for fall risk on admission to the hospital,
       transfer from another unit, and once a shift using the Hendrich
       Fall Risk Assessment Tool.
   B. Identify patient's fall risk by assessing each of the following
       evidence-based risk factors and scoring the risk points.
   C. When risk score is 3 or above, document the patient's risk score on
       admission to the hospital, transfer from another unit and once a
       shift using the Hendrich Fall Risk Assessment Tool.

1. History of Falls (not a slip or trip): Has fallen within the past 3
    months, include patient falls at home, on a previous admission
    or during this admission.   +7
2. Altered elimination: Has incontinence, frequency or nocturia,
    will have or has need to get to toilet frequently or urgently,
    likely to need to void during the night, needs assistance w/
    toileting; has frequency or diarrhea.   +3
3. Confusion/disorientation: Is not able to listen and follow
    instructions; has disorganized or unrealistic thinking patterns;
    unable to follow simple instructions and retain memory; has
    poor judgment or lacks awareness of own safety risks
    limitations. Overestimates/forgets own limitations (vs.) is
    oriented to own ability.   +3

(continued)

BOX 1. *(continued)*	
4. Depression: Currently exhibits multiple symptoms of depression such as fatigue, weight loss, lethargy, insomnia, sad affect, irritability, uncontrollable crying. Has feelings of hopelessness. Admits to being downhearted or blue.	+4
5. Dizziness/vertigo: Has orthostatic changes related to side effects of medications or medical condition:	+3
6. Nonadaptive mobility/generalized weakness: Has an unsteady gait, uses assistive devices or needs assistance; uses crutches/cane/walker or furniture as ambulatory aid; has generalized weakness or decreased mobility in lower extremities.	+2
7. Poor judgment: Lacks safety awareness, overestimates own limitations. Needs assistance to transfer or to get out of bed but still reports independence. Needs walker or crutches to ambulate but continues to use furniture to stabilize.	+3

TABLE 7.1   Types of Risk Factors

Extrinsic: External risk factors.
- Environment—wet floors, steps.
- Unstable furnishings—bedside table, step stool.
- No footwear, inappropriate footwear.
- Unsafe activity related to IV pole or other equipment.
- Poor lighting.
- Inadequate handrail support.
- Low toilet seat.
- Wheels on beds or chairs unlocked.

Intrinsic[7]/anticipated physiological[24]: Internal risk factors that result in a decreased level of adaptation by an individual.
- Recent history of falls (not slip/trip).
- Altered elimination (incontinence, nocturia, frequency).
- Confusion/Disorientation.
- Non-adaptive mobility/Generalized weakness.
- Depression.
- Dizziness/Vertigo.
- Poor judgment.

Intrinsic[7]/unanticipated physiological[24]: Unforeseeable if no previous history is present and no risk factors are identified from physical/functional assessment.
- Drop attacks.
- Cardiac arrhythmias.
- Seizure.
- Transient Ischemic Attack (TIA) or Cerebral Vascular Accident (CVA).
- Drug reactions/side effects.
- Syncope.
- Pathological fracture of hip.

FALL RISK ASSESSMENT

Well researched fall risk assessment tools provide a frame of reference to enhance the predictability of a fall. The use of a standard fall risk assessment tool establishes a consistent method for assessment and a basis for care planning. It also provides a format for the clear communication of risk prediction to all caregivers[8]. No fall risk assessment tool can successfully predict all falls. Fall risk assessment must include a general health history, as well as physical and functional assessment. The best approach to fall prevention is astute observation, clinical nursing judgment, and critical thinking skills combined with an evidence-based fall risk assessment tool.

Hendrich's Fall Risk Assessment Tool was chosen from the literature for this protocol based on the tool's sensitivity and spec-

TABLE 7.2 Risk Assessment Tool						
HENDRICH FALL RISK-ASSESSMENT TOOL						
Date						
Shift						
FALL RISK FACTOR ASSESSMENT Points						
Recent history of falls (not slip/trip) +7						
Altered elimination (incontinence, nocturia, frequency) +3						
Confusion/disorientation +3						
Depression +4						
Dizziness/vertigo +3						
Poor mobility/generalized weakness +2						
Poor judgement: (if not confused) +3						
Other:						
FINAL RISK SCORE =	SCORE	SCORE	SCORE	SCORE	SCORE	SCORE

Note: From A. Hendrich, *Falls, Immobility, and Restraints: A resource Manual* (pp. 9–17), 1996, St. Louis, MO. Mosby. Copyright 1996. Reprinted with permission.

ificity as well as other utilization factors[22]. (See Table 7.2 for Hendrich's Tool). The tool includes the following six significant risk factors: recent history of falls (not slip/trip), altered elimination, confusion/disorientation, depression, dizziness/vertigo, and non-adaptive mobility/generalized weakness, and poor judgment. Cancer diagnosis was a risk factor identified in Hendrich's[8] 1995 study, but was not included in this tool as it was not supported in a more recent unpublished study[23]. Ongoing evaluation led members of the fall prevention project team at BMC to split out poor judgment as a separate risk factor from confusion. Poor judgment was separated from confusion as a measure of clarifying the nurse's need to clearly differentiate those persons who overestimate their own self-care ability or limitations.

History of Falls

History of falls is frequently cited in the literature as a risk factor contributing to falls[8,24,25]. Using logistical regression methodology, Hendrich[8] found recent history of falls to be the most significant risk factor in the studied populations. Morse[24] states that once the patient has fallen, he or she is likely to fall a second time and under similar circumstances. History of falls can be assessed by asking the patient and family if the patient has ever fallen, when the fall occurred, and the circumstances surrounding the fall. Further questioning about associated symptoms, such as dizziness, weakness, and loss of consciousness associated with the event, can supplement the nursing assessment.

Altered Elimination

Patient fall data also suggests that elimination is often the number one related activity when a patient falls[8,16]. Rainville's study[26] reported that over half of falls occurred while the patient was using or attempting to use the commode, urinal, or bathroom. Barbieri's study[16] reported that 52% of patient falls occurred when patients attempted to void independently.

Elimination patterns can be assessed by asking the patient specific questions such as: "Once you feel the need to go to the bathroom, how long can you wait?" "Do you ever lose urine and get wet?" "Do you ever soil yourself?" "How many times do you go to the bathroom during the day?" "How many times do you get up during the night to go to the bathroom?[27]"

Confusion/Disorientation

Confusion may be intermittent or continuous in nature determined by its etiology. Hernandez and Miller[28] found patients with the diagnosis of dementia accounted for 77% of the falls in their sample. Berryman[17] reported that those patients who had periodic intervals of confusion and disorientation were more likely to fall. Schultz[29] found that lack of safety awareness was predictive of falls.

One aspect of confusion and orientation can be assessed with recall and orientation questions. A common recall test requires the nurse to name three objects (book, table, floor) and have the patient repeat those items immediately, and again in a few minutes. Orientation can be validated by asking "Where are you now?" (city, state, building, etc.), and "What day (season, month, or year) is it?[30]"

Depression

Manifestations of depression, such as difficulty with thinking or diminished concentration, predispose the individual to a fall[31]. Assessment of depression includes asking the patient if he/she feels downhearted or blue. Be alert to the fact that depressed patients will often answer questions with the statement, "I don't know.[27]" Spellbring[19] noted that when focusing on a life crisis, the depressed patient often neglects aspects of personal care and safety. Therefore, patients' appearance and personal grooming practices are considered when assessing for depression.

Dizziness /Vertigo

Dizziness/vertigo might occur as a side effect of medications or medical condition. Reassessment of medications, specifically diuretics, pain medications, barbiturates, hypnotics, and tranquilizers needs to be ongoing[16]. Nursing assessment incorporates asking the patient if he/she has ever felt dizzy on position change. Blood pressure is monitored for orthostatic changes on admission, and with each significant revision of the medication regime or treatment. If systolic blood pressure drops 20 mm Hg or more from lying to a standing position, the potential for hypotensive-related falls can be anticipated[17].

Nonadaptive Mobility/Generalized Weakness

Problems with mobility or weakness are reported repeatedly in patients who fall: for example, Tinetti[32] found impaired mobility to be a strong predictor for falls. Assessment of mobility by the "get up and go test" includes observing the patient rise from a chair, walk 10 feet, turn around and return to the chair[33]. Difficulties in ambulation, unsteadiness on one's feet, or postural sway are thus noted. The patient is asked if he/she uses assistive devices or specific techniques to ambulate at home, such as holding furniture for support and balance.

Poor Judgment

Judgment can be assessed by giving the patient hypothetical situations, such as: "The telephone is ringing but it is across the room and you can't reach it, what would you do?" or simply, "What would you do if you needed to get up to go to the bathroom?" Schultz[29] describes poor judgment as someone who "needs assistance to transfer or to get out of bed but still reports independence" or "needs walker or crutches to ambulate but continues to use furniture to stabilize."

Other Risk Factors

Risk assessment tools should be utilized as a frame of reference to enhance predictability of potential falls and selection of related prevention strategies. However, the nurse should supplement the listed risk factors on the tool with information that is specific to a patient or a particular patient population. Hendrich[7] includes an additional category of "other" to communicate nurses' physical/functional assessment of unique risk factors such as polypharmacy, sedation, or excessive blood loss. These factors in turn may clarify other noted risks.

All falls have a cause and many, if not most, are preventable[24]. Assessment must be ongoing, as fluctuations in acuity and severity may result in variance of a patient's fall risk[16]. Accurate, vigilant assessment on admission, every shift, and with any significant change in condition is considered the best approach to identifying patients who need risk related interventions. At Baystate Medical Center, a flow diagram is posted on every nursing unit to remind nursing personnel of the importance of ongoing risk factor identification. (See Figure 7.1 for flow diagram.)

FALL-PREVENTION INTERVENTIONS

The interventions found in this protocol could be classified into five categories: (a) approaches to reduce environmental hazards, (b) methods to compensate for functional limitations, (c) education to increase patient/family involvement, (d) activities to increase staff awareness of fall risk factors, and (e) patient targeted risk-related interventions. The first 3 categories are considered to be level 1 interventions, and constitute a minimum standard of care for all patients. Level 2 interventions are suggested for patients identified as high risk using the Hendrich Fall Risk Assessment Tool (score of 3 or above) and includes all 5 intervention categories. (See Box 2 for list of level 1 and level 2 interventions.)

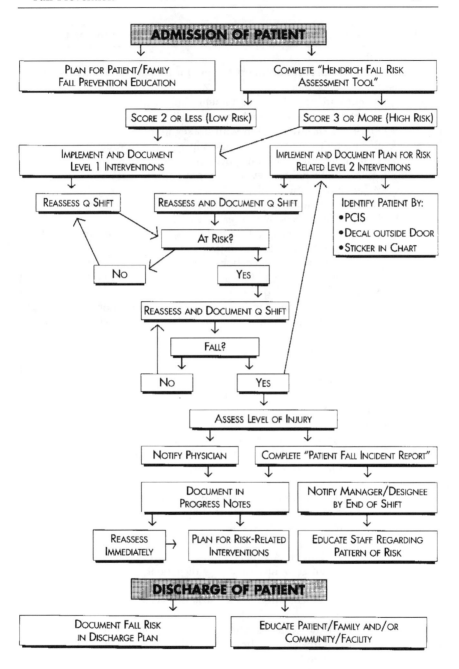

FIGURE 7.1   **Fall-prevention program flow chart.**

BOX 2.   Nursing Standard of Practice Protocol: Prevention of Falls

I. Interventions
  A. Level 1. Fall prevention interventions for all patients regardless of risk.
    1. Orient patient to the environment.
    2. Maintain call bell in reach; ensure patient is able to use.
    3. Place bed in low position with brakes locked.
    4. Ensure footwear are fitted, non-slip and used properly.
    5. Determine safest side rail position.
    6. Utilize night light on evening, night shift.
    7. Wipe spills immediately.
    8. Arrange furniture/objects safely, remove unneeded furniture.
    9. Place patient needs within easy reach.
    10. Ensure adequate handrails in bathroom, patients room and in hall.
    11. Assist with elimination as appropriate.
    12. Evaluate effects of medications that predispose patient to falls.
    13. Assist with exercise and/or have PT assess for mobility/safety.
    14. Monitor all patients q1 hour.
    15. Educate patient and family regarding fall prevention strategies.
  B. Level 2. Fall prevention interventions for patients at risk; score 3 or above.
    1. Identify patient as fall risk with identifiers as follows:
      a. In computerized information system, kardex or care plan.
      b. Fall risk sticker on chart.
      c. Fall risk decal outside patient room.
    2. Risk related interventions.
      a. History of Falls.
        i. Plan for care based on patient's fall history/previous pattern.
        ii. Utilize protective measures to prevent injury.
        iii. Utilize bed/chair-exit alarms.
      b. Altered elimination.
        i. Plan individualized schedule for voiding.
        ii. Obtain bedside commode if appropriate.
      c. Confusion/disorientation.
        i. Relocate patient for better visibility.
        ii. Maintain close supervision.
        iii. Encourage family to stay with patient.
        iv. Utilize bed-exit alarms.
        v. Request consults to Geriatric or Psychiatric APN.
      d. Depression.
        i. Evaluate patient's ability to interpret information given.
        ii. Reinforce activity limits and safety precautions to patient and family.
      e. Dizziness/Vertigo.
        i. Monitor orthostatic blood pressures.   *(continued)*

BOX 2. *(continued)*

ii. Instruct patient to:
      ◊ rise from lying to sitting position slowly.
      ◊ dangle before walking.
      ◊ perform ankle pumping in sitting position before
        walking.
      ◊ sit down immediately if feeling dizzy.
  f. Nonadaptive mobility/generalized weakness.
    i. Request consult to physical therapy.
    ii. Ensure adequate exercise to strengthen muscles.
    iii. Assist patient with ambulation.

Approaches to Reduce Environmental Hazards

Fourteen percent of all patient falls are related to environmental factors[24]. Seemingly insignificant environmental hazards may be easily overlooked by nursing personnel. The frailer a person is, the more susceptible he/she is to even minor hazards[34]. For example, an elderly patient may have access to the call bell, but arthritic changes or poor eyesight may inhibit ability to activate the call system. A soft-touch, breath-activated, or a handheld bell may be used by patients who have difficulty with standard call equipment. A list of interventions to reduce environmental hazards, such as locking wheels and assuring proper lighting, serve as a reminder to the nursing team to proactively reduce risks.

Methods to Compensate for Functional Limitations

Patients who score at high risk for falls using the tool may have diminished functional ability due to existing chronic disabilities, or iatrogenic illness resulting from medical treatment. Arthritis, sensory deficits, and altered urinary patterns are some common disabilities experienced during the aging process. Iatrogenic illnesses can occur as a result of prescribed treatments by health care workers[35]. During hospitalization, mobility limitations, intravenous therapy, Foley catheters, medications, and other therapies or treatments induce acute changes in function, which in turn places patients at high risk. Because the elderly person has a diminished ability to compensate for change, the nurse must be proactive in assisting patients to adapt.

Education to Increase Patient/Family Involvement

The basis of prevention is to provide older persons and their families with information on fall-prevention strategies. Patient education, based on nursing assessment, is recommended for all patients and families early in their hospital stay and again at the time of discharge. Determining the patient's ability to learn begins at the time of admission assessment, and continues during the routine fall assessment. Not all patients are able to participate in fall prevention education, however. Identification of those patients who are unable or not ready to learn is the first step in planning patient education. Changes in cognitive status such as delirium, dementia or depression can inhibit the patient's readiness to learn[36]. Other factors such as pain, anxiety, sleep disturbances, poor hearing and vision, and altered urinary function need to be considered before addressing fall prevention. A patient education handout is recommended to reinforce teaching (see Figure 7.2).

Activities to Increase Staff Awareness of Fall Risk Factors

Identification of the patient's risk is communicated to the health care team. The protocol suggests that once a nurse identifies a patient to be at high risk for falls, an individualized plan should be implemented. Clear, standardized documentation of risk factors, and both universal and risk-specific interventions should occur at time of admission, transfer from another unit, and when the patient's condition changes. (See Figure 2 for documentation sheet.) This protocol suggests that the patient's risk be identified by placing a standard fall-prevention decal outside the room, and a sticker on the chart. At Baystate Medical Center communication of the patient's risk is added to the nursing data in a computerized information system. Similar information could be added to a nursing care plan or kardex.

DON'T LET A FALL GET YOU DOWN!!

- If you fall while in the hospital you may suffer an injury and your recovery will be slowed.
- It is more common to fall in situations that are strange and unfamiliar to you. In addition, noise, light, scheduling of tests, or other factors may make it more difficult for you to rest, leaving you tired and more vulnerable to falling.

SUGGESTIONS FOR PREVENTING FALLS

- Move your joints and muscles as much as possible.
- Walk close to the wall, use a railing to support yourself.
- When recommended, use assistive devices like a walker/cane or wheechair.
- Hold onto the handrail in the bathroom.
- Get up slowly from bed or chair to prevent dizziness. Your health care team will be happy to assist you.
- Wear non-skid footwear. Avoid using loose fitting shoes such as flip/flops.
- Report spills or hazardous conditions to your health care team.
- Have necessary items within reach: phone, tissue, water pitcher, call bell, and anything else you need.
- Use your call bell for assistance to get things that are beyond your reach.
- Call for assistance when you need help with toileting.

IF YOU FALL:

✓ **Try to stay calm.**
✓ **Don't leap up, you may be injured. Stay where you are and wait for help to arrive.**
✓ **Call for help. Use the call light if possible or call out for help.**

By being aware of your surroundings and the guidelines above:
YOU CAN PREVENT A FALL!!!

FIGURE 7.2   Fall-prevention patient education flyer.

Patient-Targeted Risk-Related Interventions

A standard fall-prevention program is most effective when interventions are individualized[8]. When a recent history of falling is identified, interventions are indicated that reduce or compensate for the underlying cause. Patients who exhibit signs of "sundowning" may be more at risk to fall in the evening. Keeping the room brightly lit or asking a family member to visit at that time may reduce the risk. In contrast, those with Parkinson's disease may be at greater risk in early morning, or when experiencing "wear-ing-off" effects of their medication. In anticipation of stiffness and decreased mobility, the nursing personnel may provide additional assistance at these times. Patients with confusion and altered mobility may try to go to the toilet unaided. Diuretics may cause an individual to rush to the toilet. A program of scheduled toileting may help prevent falls in these situations.

Electronic warning devices (bed and chair alarms) are widely suggested as an intervention in prevention of falls[8,37–42]. Alarm systems are designed to alert nursing staff that patients who require assistance with mobility are leaving the bed or chair. Indications for alarm systems include those patients with a history of falls, unsafe bed mobility, cognitive deficits, confusion, or inability to use the call bell. The efficacy of an alarm system depends on effective technology, and the response time of nursing staff[39]. A program of staff, patient, and family education that includes rationale for using the alarm, and how to set up and operate the alarm, is recommended to enhance the effectiveness of the intervention.

Restraints

Historically, restraints have been perceived as a method to prevent falls. Restraint use has not been included as a fall-prevention intervention in this protocol, as use of restraints is recognized, in actuality, to contribute to patients' risk for falls and related injuries[43]. The Joint Commission on Accreditation of Healthcare Organizations (JACHO) 1998 Standards[44] recommends creating an environment to reduce restraint use by using preventive or alternative strategies. Alternatives to restraints such as close, frequent observation are essential and may be accomplished by moving the patient closer to the nurse's station; enlisting family or friends or volunteers as companions, and using electronic warning devices[43].

OUTCOME INDICATORS

Fall-prevention programs are thought to commonly fail due to inadequate interventions and insufficient monitoring or tracking[7]. A rigid rather than flexible approach to program development and implementation may fail to identify the unique needs of specialized patient populations (e.g.. neurology; cardiovascular; oncology). A method for auditing current, unit-specific practice and for collecting and using postfall data are essential for continuous quality improvement. Relevant evidence can then be provided to nursing staff so that they understand the current level and impact of their own practice.

Key elements used to track the progress of a fall-prevention program include fall rate and injury index. Reporting fall rates, rather than the number of falls, is a more accurate measure of improvement. Such a rate is calculated by the number of falls divided by patient days times 1000[32,35]. These rates can vary by type of institution, patient acuity and clinical service. Published fall rates, as well as institutional and unit-specific data, can serve as a benchmark for measuring improvement as the program is implemented.

Classification of severity of injury is also an important quality indicator. The injury index is calculated by number of injuries divided by number of falls times 100. Hendrich[7] suggests that injuries be categorized into 5 classes: (1) no injury, (2) minor injury, (3) moderate injury, (4) major injury and (5) death (See Table 7.3 for injury classi-

TABLE 7.3   Injury Classifications

Class	Injury
Class I: No injury	No visible evidence of any physical injury (e.g., bruise, abrasion, reddened area.)
Class II: Minor injury	A small scrape, abrasion, or bruise that heals without treatment in a few days.
Class III: Moderate injury	A suspected bone injury requiring an x-ray but with no evidence of fracture. A laceration that requires suturing and medical treatment. An IV that infiltrates after the fall requiring treatment.
Class IV: Major Injury	A confirmed fracture of any bone or head injury.
Class V: Death	A direct result of a fall event. May occur a few hours, days, or months later as a result of complications.

Note: Adapted from A. Hendrich, *Falls, Immobility, and Restraints: A resource Manual* (pp. 9–17), 1996, St. Louis, MO. Mosby.

fications.) Injury rates (class 2–5) in acute care have been reported to range from 20% to 30%[45]. Serious injuries (classes 4 and 5) have been reported to range from 2% to 6%[24]. Therefore, baseline data can include the following, reported by both overall hospital and individual unit: fall rate, index of all injuries (classes 2–5), and index of severe injuries (classes 4 and 5) (See Box 3 for outcome indicators).

When evaluating the success of fall-prevention interventions, it is important to review both fall rate and injury index. In many cases, the fall rate will increase with the implementation of a fall-prevention program due to heightened awareness, that is, conscious raising may lead to increased fall reporting. With this phenomenon there may also be a decrease in the injury index related to the increased reporting of minor falls that did not result in injury.

The location, time, and circumstances of a fall, as well as patient risk factors, are tracked. This information should help in identifying high-volume or peak fall periods. These peaks can be reviewed to suggest adjustments in schedules or routines and to prioritize staff education needs. At Baystate Medical Center, a unit poster is updated quarterly in narrative and graphic dis-

---

BOX 3.   **Nursing Standard Of Practice Protocol: Prevention of Falls**

I. OUTCOME INDICATORS:
Reported quarterly by individual nursing units and overall inpatient units.
  A. Calculate the following for the overall hospital and individual unit/service:
    1. Fall rate: Number of falls divided by patient days times 1000.
    2. Injury index: Number of injuries divided by number of falls times 100.
    3. Major injury index: Number of severe injuries (fractures, head injury or death) divided by number of falls times 100.
  B. Shift and time that majority of falls occurred.
  C. Utilization and effectiveness of the risk assessment tool.
  D. Position of side rails or use of restraints.
  E. Percentage of falls by specific risk factors.
  F. Percentage of falls that were extrinsic, intrinsic or unanticipated.
  G. Utilization and effectiveness of bed exit alarms.
  H. Utilization and effectiveness of other specific targeted interventions related to fall risk factors.
  I. Relationship of side rail position to the severity of injury.
  J. Evaluation of effectiveness of surveillance personnel (sitters).

plays. Specific information includes fall rates in acute care cited in the literature; current unit fall rate and injury index including changes over time; peak times of falls; and patient location and activity at the time of the fall. Unit-specific data is combined with other unit-related information on falls to enable staff to evaluate the quality of their practice.

Documenting use of protective devices such as side rails or alarm systems is important in order to evaluate the effectiveness of the equipment and the appropriateness of the initial application. Historically, side rails have been considered to be a protective device intended to keep patients in bed. A relationship may exist between position of side rail and severity of injury. Clearly, caregivers can learn much from their own data to enhance fall prevention interventions.

Recording and analyzing the risk factors present at the time of the fall is helpful in identifying the need for additional interventions specific to that risk factor. For example, if the majority of falls reported on a cardiac unit have the common risk of dizziness, the staff can research and target interventions specific to that problem. Trends may also identify common characteristics of patients who continue to fall despite routine interventions thus facilitating further creative problem solving.

Finally, a fall-prevention "program" is an innovation aimed at producing quality care. To succeed, however, individual components of the innovation or program (e.g., risk assessment tool and interventions) must be accurately and consistently implemented. Careful and continuous monitoring is needed to assess the integrity of the innovation[46] by providing detailed evalutation of the actual process of care. Feedback from these evaluations, along with outcome data, provides useful information to nurses and institutional stakeholders in order to continuously improve the program.

CONCLUSIONS

A fall can significantly alter the course of hospitalization and impact the quality of life of a hospitalized elder. Early identification of potential falls, using an evidence-based risk assessment tool and critical evaluation of the usefulness of related interventions, are essential for effective fall prevention. A nursing standard of practice protocol, combined with good nursing judgment, provides nurses the opportunity to have a direct impact on the quality of care of the hospitalized elderly.

ACKNOWLEDGMENTS

Many have supported and contributed to the development of this Fall-Prevention Protocol. Mary Brunell, MS, RN, VP for Nursing and Margaret Burns, PhD, RN, Director of Medical-Surgical and Critical Care Nursing have administratively supported the project throughout its development. Particular credit goes to members of the Baystate Medical Center Fall Prevention Quality Improvement Project Team: Penny Begley, RN, Maura Brennan, MD, Catherine Buelow, RPT, Michael Davis, RN, Monica Dubiel, RN, Sally Green, JD, Eileen Grunwald, MS, RN, Lynn Guidi, RN, Patricia Humiston, RN, Theresa Oh, RN, Dianne Parelli, PTA, and Carol Strobelberger, RN. Thanks also to Maureen Sullivan from Graphic Design. Finally, our appreciation is extended to Ann Hendrich for her fall prevention research and for allowing us to adapt her model for this protocol.

This project was supported by the Baystate Health Systems Insurance Company Risk Management Grant.

REFERENCES

[1] Nevitt MC, Cumming SR, Kidd S, Black D. Risk factors for recurrent nonsyncopal falls: A prospective study. *JAMA.* 1989;18:2663–2668.
[2] Baraff LJ. Practice guideline for the ED management of falls in community dwelling elderly persons. *Ann Emerg Med.* 1997;30:480–492.
[3] Langlois JA, Smith GS, Baker SP, Langley JD. International comparisons of injury mortality in the elderly: Issues and differences between New Zealand and the United States. *Intl J Epidemiolo.* 24:136–43, 1995.

[4]   Marottoli RA, Berkman LF, Cooney LF. Decline in physical function following hip fracture. *J Am Geriatr Soc.* 1992;40:861–866.

[5]   Morgan V, Mathison J, Rice J, Clemmer D. Hospital falls: A persistent problem. *Am J Pub Health.* 1985;75:775–777.

[6]   Maciorowski L, Munro B, Dietrick-Gallagher M, McNew C, Shepperd-Hinkel E, Wanich C. A review of the patient fall literature. *J Qual Ass.* 1988;3(1):18–27.

[7]   Hendrich A. *Falls, Immobility and Restraints: A Resource Manual.* St Louis, MO: Mosby; 1996.

[8]   Hendrich A, Nyhuis A, Kippenbrock T, Soja ME. Hospital falls: Development of a predictive model for clinical practice. *Appl Nurs Res.* 1995;8(3):129–139.

[9]   Cohen L, Guin P. Implementation of a patient fall prevention program. *J Neurosci Nurs.* 1991;23(5):315–319.

[10] Morse JM, Morse RM, Tylko SJ. Development of a scale to identify the fall prone patient. *Can J Aging.* 1989;8:366–377.

[11] Schmid N. Reducing patient falls: A research-based comprehensive fall prevention program. *Mili Med.* 1990;155:202–207.

[12] Hogue, CC. Managing falls: The current bases for practice. In *Key Aspects of Elder Care.* New York: Springer Publishing Co.; 1992; p. 41.

[13] Morse JM. Nursing research on patient falls in health care institutions. *Ann Rev Nurs Res.* 1993;11:299–316.

[14] Kilpack V, Boehm J, Smith N, Mudge B. Using research based interventions to decrease patient falls. *Appl Nurs Res.* 1991;4(2):50–56.

[15] Jenkin J, Reynolds B, Swiech K. Patient falls in the acute care setting: Identifying risk factors. *Nurs Res.* 1986;35:215–219.

[16] Barbieri E. Patient falls are not patient accidents. *J Gerontol Nurs.* 1983;9:165–173.

[17] Berryman E, Gaskin D, Jones A, Tolley F, MacMullen J. Point by point: Predicting elders' falls. *Geriatr Nurs.* 1989;July/August:199–201.

[18] Fife DD, Solomon P, Stanton M. A risk/falls program: Code orange for success. *Nurs Management.* 1984;15(11):50–53.

[19] Spellbring AM, Gannon ME, Kleckner T, Conway K. Improving safety for hospitalized elderly. *J Gerontol Nurs.* 1988;14(2):31–37.

[20] Tack K, Ulrich B, Kehr C. Patient falls: Profile for prevention. *J Neurosci Nurs.* 1987;19(2):83–89.

[21] MacAvoy S, Skinner T, and Hines M. Fall risk assessment tool. *Appl Nurs Res.* 1996;9:213–218.

[22] Stetler CB, Morsi D, Rucki S, Broughton S, Corrigan B, Fitzgerald J,

Giuliano K, Havener P, Sheridan EA. Utilization-focused integrative reviews in a nursing service. *Appl Nurs Res.* 1998;11(4):195–206.

[23] Hendrich A. Personal communication, 1997.

[24] Morse, J. *Preventing Patient Falls.* Thousand Oaks, CA: Sage; 1997.

[25] Tinetti ME, Speechley M, Ginter SF. Risk factors for falls prevention among elderly persons living in the community. *New Engl J Med.* 1988;319(26):1701–1707.

[26] Rainville N. Effect of an implemented fall prevention program. *Qual Rev bull.* 1984;9:287–291.

[27] Miller C. *Nursing Care of Older Adults: Theory and Practice* (2nd ed.) Philadelphia: Lippincott; 1995.

[28] Hernandez M, Miller J. How to reduce falls. *Geriatr Nurs.* 1986;March/April:97–102.

[29] Shultz A. Personal communication, 1997.

[30] Folstein MF, Folstein SR, McHugh PR. Mini-Mental State: A practical method for grading the cognitive state of patients for the clinician. *J Psychiatr Res.* 1975;12:189–198.

[31] Eliopoulos C. *Manual of Gerontological Nursing.* St Louis, MO: Mosby; 1995.

[32] Tinetti ME, Williams TF, Mayewski R. Fall risk index for elderly patients based on number of chronic disabilities. *Am J Med.* 1986;80:429–434.

[33] Mathias S, Nayak, US, Isaacs B. Balance in elderly patients: The get up and go test. *Arch Phys Med Rehab.* 1986;67:387–389.

[34] Tinnetti ME, Speechley M. Prevention of falls among the elderly. *New Engl J Med.* 1989;320:1055–1059.

[35] Ross JER. Iatrogenesis in the elderly: Contributors to falls. *J Gerontol Nurs.* 1991;17(9):19–23.

[36] Foreman M, Fletcher K, Mion L, Simon L. Assessing cognitive function. *Geriatr Nurs.* 1996;17:228–232.

[37] Cutillo-Schmitter T A, Rovner B, Shmuely Y, Bawduniak I. Formulating treatment partnerships with patients and their families. *J Gerontol Nurs.* 1996;22(6):23–36.

[38] Braun JV, Lipson S. *Toward a Restraint-Free Environment.* Baltimore, MD: Health Professions Press, 1993.

[39] Tideiksaar R, Finer CF Maby J. Falls prevention: The efficacy of a bed alarm system in an acute-care setting. *Mt Sinai J Med.* 1993;60:522–527.

[40] Morton D. Five years of fewer falls. *Am J Nurs.* 1989;89:204–205.

[41] Innes E. Maintaining fall prevention. *Qual Rev Bull.* 1985;11:217–221.

[42] Hendrich, AL. An effective unit-based fall prevention plan. *J Nurs Qual Ass.* 1988;3:28–36.

[43] Mion L, Strumpf N. Use of physical restraints in the hospital setting: Implications for the nurse. *Geriatr Nurs.* 1994;15:127–131.

[44] Joint Commission on Accreditation of Healthcare Organizations. *1998 Accreditation Standards.* Oakbrook Terrace, IL: 1998; p. 95.

[45] Rhode JM, Myers AH, Vlahov D. Variation in risk for falls by clinical department: Implications for prevention. *Infect Control Hosp Epidemiology* 1990;11(10):21–22.

[46] Stetler C, Creer E, Effken J. Evaluating a redesign program: Challenges and opportunities. In K.elly K, (Ed), *Series on Nursing Administration* (Vol. 8). St. Louis: Mosby Year Book, 1996:231–243.

Chapter 8

PREVENTING PRESSURE ULCERS

Denise M. Kresevic, Mary D. Naylor, and the NICHE Faculty

EDUCATIONAL OBJECTIVES

On completion of this chapter, the reader should be able to:
1. Identify risk factors associated with the development of pressure ulcers.
2. Describe assessment parameters associated with the prevention of pressure ulcers.
3. Describe interventions to maintain and improve skin integrity.
4. Define strategies to avoid or minimize pressure, friction, and shearing of skin.
5. Identify patient outcomes expected from the implementation of this practice protocol.

Pressure ulcers, the most common iatrogenic illness in health care, most frequently occur in persons who are immobile or elderly with fragile skin. An extensive study of pressure ulcers in acute care facilities revealed an incidence from 3% to 28%[1]. Most facil-

Reproduced from Kresevic, DM, Naylor, M. Preventing pressure ulcers through use of protocols in a mentored nursing model. *Geriatric Nursing, 16,* 225–229. With permission from Mosby-Year Book, Inc.

ities report rates of over 9%[2]. Pressure ulcers are associated with significant complications, including cellulitis, osteomyelitis, and sepsis, and substantial costs and suffering[3]. Patient with pressure ulcers have increased costs of care and lengths of stays[1]. In one study the mean length of stay was five times longer for patients with pressure ulcers than for those without[1].

RISK FACTORS

Most pressure ulcers can be prevented; however, even the most proactive and diligent nursing care may not prevent the development of pressure ulcers in some high-risk persons[4]. Several factors contribute to the development of pressure ulcers, and a combination of risk factors, rather than one single factor, place the patient at the greatest risk for skin breakdown[5,6].

Risk factors for skin breakdown are immobility, tissue friability, poor nutrition, incontinence, impaired cognitive ability, and a decreased ability to respond to the environment[7]. These risk factors are included in widely used bedside assessment instruments. The Norton Scale and the Braden Scale identify specific risk factors for pressure ulcers and rate their severity. Many hospitals have incorporated these assessment tools into admission forms and daily flowsheets. Those patients at high risk are candidates for nursing interventions essential to reduce the risk of tissue breakdown. For patients with existing pressure sores, treatment, evaluation, and monitoring are needed to prevent (1) the progression of existing wounds, (2) the development of new breakdown, and (3) complications, such as infections.

TEACHING NURSES SKIN CARE PROTOCOLS

In 1992 the U.S. Public Health Service published nursing care guidelines on skin care[3,8]. At about the same time researchers supported by the John A. Hartford Foundation began investigating functional decline in hospitalized elders. One area of functional decline, was skin breakdown. As a part of the study on prevention of functional decline a preventative and restorative skin care protocol was implemented at the University Hospitals of Cleveland. This protocol was developed by geriatric clinical experts as part of the Hartford Study (Box 1).

Implementation of these protocols provided the opportunity to explore educational strategies to assist nurses to learn skin care protocols and enhance their clinical practice of these skills. Nurses at the University Hospitals of Cleveland volunteered to participate in an educational mentoring program. Implementation of the skin care protocol began with an educational program that used didactic teaching, combined with mentoring, to teach a myriad of skills.

The program goals were to help nurses develop skills in the early identification of risk factors, the prevention of skin breakdown, and the management of pressure ulcers. Working with the clinical nurse specialist at the bedside of patients provided the nurses a unique learning opportunity. It was expected that nurses completing the program would not only develop individual skills but also function as clinical resource persons, role models, and mentors to other nurses on their unit and other nursing units. After completing this program these nurses did agree to function as resources to their peers.

Before the educational program began, the clinical nurse specialist and the medical director of the unit developed the skin care protocol and flowsheets to monitor skin care. The pilot resource program used a didactic learning session that included assessment and management of pressure ulcers based on the U.S. Public Health Service guidelines. This workshop was followed by a bedside mentoring experience. The mentoring experience included the use of a skills checklist (Box 2). Opportunities included bedside assessment of risk factors for pressure ulcers, assessment of wounds, treatment of wounds (including cleaning agents, packing, and debriding), patient teaching, and documentation. Resource nurses assigned themselves as primary nurses to patients they admitted to the hospital. All patients were then assessed daily, using skin care protocol, from admission to discharge by the primary nurse and clinical nurse specialist. Assessments, documentation, and patient and family teaching were done by the primary

---

BOX 1.   Protocol for Prevention of Pressure Sores*

GOAL: Protect against the adverse effects of external mechanical forces: Pressure, friction, and shear.

I.   GENERAL GUIDELINES

   A.   Any person in bed assessed to be at risk for pressure ulcers should be repositioned at least every 2 hours if consistent with patient goals. A written schedule for systematically turning and repositioning the individual should be used.

   B.   For individuals in bed, positioning devices (such as pillows or foam wedges) should be used to keep bony prominences (such as knees or ankles) from direct contact with one another, according to a written plan.

   C.   Individuals in bed who are completely immobile should have a care plan that includes that use of devices that totally relieve pressure on the heels, most commonly by raising the heels off the bed. Do not use donut-type devices.

   D.   When the side-lying position is used in bed, avoid positioning directly on the trochanter.

   E.   Maintain the head of the bed at the lowest degree of elevation consistent with medical conditions and other restrictions. Limit the amount of time the head of the bed is elevated.

   F.   Use lifting devices, such as a trapeze or bed linen, to move (rather than drag) individuals in bed who cannot assist during transfers and position changes.

   G.   Any person assessed to be at risk for pressure ulcers should be placed when lying in bed on a pressure-reducing device, such as foam, static air, alternating air, gel, or water mattresses.

   H.   Any person at risk for a pressure ulcer should avoid uninterrupted sitting in any chair or wheelchair. The individual should be repositioned, shifting the points under pressure, at least every hour or be put back to bed if consistent with overall patient management goals. Individuals who are able should be taught to shift weight every 15 minutes.

   I.   For chair-bound persons, the use of a pressure-reducing pad, such as those made of foam, gel, air, or a combination, is indicated. Do not use donut-type devices.

II.   ASSESSMENT PARAMETERS

   A.   For all patients, request information about skin care regimen from prehospital setting.

   B.   On admission, identify as at risk for pressure ulcers any elderly patient who has either an impaired nutrition status or an impaired ability to move as a result of disease condition or treatment.

   C.   Assess all at-risk patients by using a standardized assessment

(continued)

BOX 1. *(continued)*

instrument. The Braden Scale, for example, takes roughly 10 minutes to administer.

D. Document risk factors, skin assessment, and plan for prevention and treatment, including a schedule for using assessment scale and care strategies.

III. CARE STRATEGIES
  A. Prevention
    1. Educate patients, families, and caregivers on the prevention of pressure ulcers. This should include:
      a. Etiology of and risk factors for pressure ulcers.
      b. Risk assessment tools and their application.
      c. Skin assessment.
      d. Selection and/or use of support surfaces.
      e. Development and implementation of an individualized program of skin care.
      f. Demonstration of positioning to reduce risk of tissue breakdown.
      g. Accurate documentation.
    2. Identify those persons responsible for pressure ulcer prevention and describe their role. Update the program on a regular basis to incorporate new information.
    3. Develop, implement, and evaluate programs using principles of adult learning. Present audience-appropriate level of information. Include built-in quality assurance standards and mechanisms.

Maintain and improve skin integrity:
    1. Using a standardized instrument and/or body chart, check skin daily, especially bony prominences, and document results.
    2. Keep skin clean and dry. Avoid hot water, strong soap, and other irritation agents, such as urine and wound drainage.
    3. Keep skin supple. Use humidifiers, moisturizers, and keep patient well hydrated (8 glasses of noncaffeinated fluid per day unless there is a fluid restriction).
    4. Do not massage skin over bony prominences.
    5. Good nutrition is important to healthy skin. Make sure patient receives adequate calories, protein, vitamin C, and zinc.
    6. Keep patient active. Movement is important in maintaining skin integrity.
    7. Document strategies implemented and their outcomes.

Avoid pressure, friction, and shearing of skin:
    1. Patients on bed rest should change, or have their position changed, every 2 hours.
    2. Use pillows or foam wedges to keep legs apart when the patient lies on side. Do not let patient lie directly on trochanter.

(continued)

BOX 1. *(continued)*

---

   3. Use pillows or other devices (not donuts) to lift heels (which
      break down easily) off bed.
   4. Use pressure-reducing mattresses and chair cushions with
      patients who cannot change position without assistance.
   5. Keep the head of the bed as low as possible, and limit the
      amount of time the head of the bed is elevated.
   6. Document strategies implemented and their outcomes.
   B. Treatment
   1. If skin impairment occurs, inspect lesion daily and document
      location, size (centimeters), stage (1–4), odor, condition of skin
      surrounding lesion, drainage.
   2. Carry out treatment plan appropriate to lesion stage[3].
   3. Educate patient, family, and caregivers on assessment,
      prevention, and treatment strategies.
IV. EXPECTED OUTCOMES
   A. Patients:
   1. Patient skin integrity will be maintained.
   2. Patients will leave the hospital with no pressure ulcers.
   3. Patients and caregivers will, at discharge, be able to identify
      risk factors for pressure ulcers and be familiar with strategies
      for assessment and prevention.
   4. Progress will be made in reversal of any existing pressure
      ulcers.
   B. Health Care Providers:
   1. Documentation of screening, processes of care, and outcomes
      will be improved.
   C. Institution:
   1. Incidence and prevalence of pressure ulcers among
      hospitalized elders will decrease.
V. FOLLOW-UP/MONITOR CONDITION
   A. Educate caregivers to continue assessment process.
   B. Show evidence of transfer of information to discharge setting.
   C. Continue to track incidence and prevalence of pressure ulcers
      among patients admitted.

---

*A more extensive protocol may be obtained by contacting the author.

---

nurse, who used the clinical nurse specialist as a mentor to validate intervention. Patients' responses to these interventions were
reviewed daily by the primary nurse in interdisciplinary rounds,
where physicians, nutritionists, physical therapists, and home care
nurses reviewed patients' needs and progress.

Most nurses who participated in the program had less than 3

BOX 2. Mentor's Assessment of Skill Mastery Demonstration

Rating

_____ 1. Verbalizes four stages of wounds based on color and depth.

_____ 2. Initiates plan of care based on individual patient's risk factors and/or stage of wound.

_____ 3. Demonstrates proper wound cleaning with appropriate agents.

_____ 4. Demonstrates proficiency in dressing selection and application.

_____ 5. Demonstrates proficiency in packing wound.

_____ 6. Demonstrates inclusive documentation of patient risk factors, wound staging, intervention, and patient response.

_____ 7. Demonstrates discussion of intervention with patient and/or family (caregiver).

Evaluating rating scale

_____ 3 Accomplished accurately with minimal direction/assistance

_____ 2 Accomplished accurately with moderate direction/assistance

_____ 1 Accomplished accurately with significant direction/assistance

_____   _____

RN signature   Date

_____   _____

Resource RN signature   Date

Follow-up plans _____

_____

_____

---

years of clinical experience; all had at least 1 year. Ten nurses completed the skin care resource program. All rated the bedside monitoring experience as the most effective strategy with which to apply knowledge and develop confidence. Working with the mentor provided the nurses the opportunity to quickly assess and intervene, while validating their didactic learning. The bedside mentoring experience, an active learning process, quickly validated assessments, interventions, patient teaching, and documentation. Participating nurses also identified that bedside mentoring allowed for efficient use of time. The mentor and the nurse provided patient care while learning. None of the patients followed up by these resource nurses had additional pressure ulcers develop, and over half of the patients had evidence of wound healing and granulation for existing wounds within the short mean length of stay of 7.4 days.

Materials to assist in the education of patients, families, and caregivers are an essential component of any skin care program to prevent tissue breakdown. At the University Hospitals of Cleveland, The U.S. Public Health Service Patient Guide "Preventing Pressure Ulcers: A Patient's Guide" is given to all patients and reviewed daily.

SUMMARY

Few conditions offer a better opportunity for nurses to have a dramatic and visible impact on quality care than skin care. Nursing interventions targeted to prevent pressure ulcers and their painful, costly complications are an expected standard of care in all care settings. Preventing pressure ulcers may be most important in the acute care setting, where previously healthy elders with acute illness, immobility, impaired appetite, and new-onset incontinence may suddenly and unexpectedly develop pressure ulcers. Often acute care nurses have not been fully cognizant of the threat that pressure ulcers can pose for acutely ill patients. Teaching nurses skills of prevention, including assessments, and interventions for this group of patients is critical. Traditional teaching methods supplemented with an innovative mentoring program and clinical protocols may be one way to accomplish this.

REFERENCES

[1] Allman RM. Pressure sores among the elderly. *N Engl J Med.* 1989;320:850–3.
[2] Andrychuk, MA Pressure ulcers: Causes, risk factors, assessment and intervention. *Orthopaed Nurs.* 1988;16(5):65–81.
[3] U.S. Department of Health and Human Services, Agency for Health Care Policy and Research, Public Health Service. *Pressure Ulcers in Adults: Prediction and Prevention.* (Clinical Practice Guideline, No. 3.) Rockville, MD: AHCPR Publication No. 92–0047, May 1992.
[4] O'Brien SP, Wind S, van Rijswijk L, Kerstein MD. Sequential biannual prevalence studies of pressure ulcers at Allegheny-Hahnemann

University Hospital. *Ostomy Wound Manage.* 1998;Mar;44(3A Suppl):78S–88S.

[5] Norton D, McLaren R, Exton-Smith AN. *An Investigation of Geriatric Nursing Problems in the Hospital.* London: National Corporation for the Care of Old People, 1962.

[6] Bergstrom N, Braden, BJ, Laguzza A, and Homan Z. The Braden Scale for predicting pressure sore risk. *Nurs Res.* 1987;36(4):205–210.

[7] Braden BJ. The relationship between stress and pressure sore formation. *Ostomy Wound Manage.* 1998;44(3A Suppl.):265–365.

[8] Bergman-Evans B, Cuddigan J, Bergstrom N. Clinical practice guidelines: Prediction and prevention of pressure ulcers, *J Gerontol Nurs.* 1994;20(9):19–26.

Chapter 9

DEPRESSION IN ELDERLY PATIENTS

Lenore H. Kurlowicz and the NICHE Faculty

EDUCATIONAL OBJECTIVES

On completion of this chapter, the reader should be able to:
1. Discuss the consequences of depression for elderly patients.
2. Identify nursing strategies for elders with depression.
3. Discuss the major risk factors for late-life depression.
4. Identify the core components of a systematic nursing assessment for depression with elderly patients.

Depression in late life is common. Nearly 5 million of the 31 million Americans aged 65 and older have depression[1]. Prevalence studies report significant rates of combined major and minor depression in various populations of older adults: community dwelling (13%), medical outpatients (24%), acute care (30%), and nursing homes (43%)[2]. Certain populations have higher levels of depressive symptoms, particularly those with more severe or chronic disabling conditions, such as those elders in acute and long-term care settings. Depression also frequently coexists with

Reproduced from Kurlowicz, LH, Nursing standard of practice protocols: Depression in elderly patients. *Geriatric Nursing, 18,* 192–200. With permission of Mosby-Year Book, Inc.

dementia, specifically Alzheimer's disease, with prevalence rates ranging from 10% to 40%[3,4]. Cognitive impairment may be a secondary symptom of depression or depression may be the result of dementia[2].

The coexistence of many physical, social, and economic problems in late life frequently impedes timely recognition and treatment of depression, with subsequent unnecessary morbidity and death[1]. A substantial number of elderly patients encountered by nurses will have clinically relevant depressive symptoms. Thus, nurses remain at the frontline in early recognition of depression and facilitation of elderly patients' access to mental health care. This chapter presents an overview of depression in elderly patients, with emphasis on age-related assessment considerations, clinical decision-making, and nursing intervention strategies for elders with depression. A standard of practice protocol for use by nurses in practice settings is also presented.

WHAT IS DEPRESSION?

In the broadest sense, depression is defined as a syndrome comprised of a constellation of affective, cognitive, and somatic or physiological manifestations[5]. Depression may range in severity from mild symptoms to more severe forms, both of which can persist over longer periods of time with negative consequences for the elderly patient. Suicidal ideation, psychotic features, especially delusional thinking, and excessive somatic concerns frequently accompany more severe depression[5]. Symptoms of anxiety may also coexist with depression in many older adults[6].

The *Diagnostic and Statistical Manual of Mental Disorders* (DSM-IV)[7] currently lists specific criteria that are necessary for a diagnosis of a major depressive disorder, the most severe form of depression, and that are frequently used as the standard by which elderly patients' depressive symptoms are counted in clinical settings[7]. Five symptoms from a list of nine (affective, cognitive, and somatic) must be present nearly every day during the same 2–week period and must represent a change from previous functioning. The nine symptoms include (1) depressed, sad, or irritable mood, (2) anhedonia or diminished pleasure in usually pleasurable people or activities, (3) feelings of worthlessness, self-reproach, or excessive guilt, (4) difficulty with thinking or diminished concentration, (5) suicidal thinking or attempts, (6) fatigue and loss of energy, (7) changes in appetite and weight, (8) disturbed sleep, and (9) psychomotor agitation or retardation. For this diagnosis, at least one of the five symptoms must include either depressed mood, by the patient's subjective account or observation of others, or markedly diminished pleasure in almost all people or activities. Concurrent medical conditions are frequently present in elderly patients and should not preclude a diagnosis of depression; indeed, there is a high incidence of comorbidity.

Elderly patients may more readily report somatic or physical symptoms than depressed mood[8]. The somatic or physical symptoms of depression, however, are often difficult to distinguish from somatic or physical symptoms associated with acute or chronic physical illnesses, especially in the hospitalized elderly patient, or the somatic symptoms that are part of common aging processes[9]. In particular, disturbed sleep may be associated with a chronic lung disease, congestive heart failure, or changes in sleeping patterns or habits. Diminished energy or increased lethargy may be caused by an acute metabolic disturbance or drug response. Therefore, a challenge for nurses in acute care hospitals and other clinical settings is to not overlook or disregard somatic or physical complaints while also "looking beyond" such complaints to assess the full spectrum of depressive symptoms in elderly patients. In elders with acute medical illnesses, somatic symptoms that persist may indicate a more serious depression, in spite of treatment of the underlying medical illness or discontinuance of a depressogenic medication[9]. Elderly patients may link their somatic or physical complaints to a depressed mood or anhedonia. Depression also may be expressed through repetitive verbalizations (e.g., calling out for help) or agitated vocalizations (e.g., screaming, yelling, or shouting), repetitive questions, expressions of unrealistic fears (e.g., fear of abandonment, being left alone), repetitive statements that something bad will happen, and repetitive health-related concerns[10].

MINOR DEPRESSION

Although major depression as defined by the DSM-IV seems to be less common among older than younger cohorts, there is evidence of a high prevalence of less severe depressive symptoms that are of clinical significance, especially in medically ill elderly patients, and for which treatment may be warranted[11]. Such depressive symptoms have been variously referred to in the literature as "minor depression," "subsyndromal depression," "dysthymic depression," "subclinical depression," "elevated depressive symptoms," and "mild depression." Minor depression is two to four times as common as major depression in older adults and is associated with increased risk of subsequent major depression and greater use of health services, as well as having a negative impact on physical and social functioning and quality of life[11–13].

COURSE OF DEPRESSION

Depression can occur for the first time in late life, or it can be part of a long-standing affective or mood disorder. Older hospitalized medically ill patients with depression are also more likely to have had a previous depression of other psychiatric illness, including alcohol abuse[14]. As in younger people, the course of depression in older adults is characterized by exacerbations, remissions, and chronicity[5]. Therefore, a wait-and-see approach with regard to treatment is not recommended.

DEPRESSION IN LATE LIFE IS SERIOUS

Research has shown that depression is associated with serious negative consequences for older adults, especially for frail elderly patients, such as those recovering from a severe medical illness or those in nursing homes. Consequences of depression include amplification of pain and disability, delayed recovery from medical illness or surgery, worsening of medical symptoms, risk of physical illness, increased health care utilization, alcoholism, cognitive impairment, worsening social impairment, protein-calorie subnutrition, and increased rates of suicide and non-suicide-related death[15]. The recent "amplification" hypothesis proposed by Katz et al.[16] stated that depression can "turn up the volume" on several aspects of physical, psychosocial, and behavioral functioning in elderly patients ultimately accelerating the course of medical illness. For elderly nursing home residents, depression is also associated with poor adjustment to the nursing home, resistance to daily care, treatment refusal, inability to participate in activities, and further social isolation[17]. Major depression can amplify cognitive impairment and functional disability in Alzheimer's disease[4].

Mortality rates by suicide are higher among elderly persons with depression than among their counterparts without depression and cannot be accounted for by sociodemographic factors or preexisting illness[18]. Although older adults account for 12% of the population, they account for 21% of suicides[19]. White men over age 80 are at greatest risk and are six times more likely to commit suicide than the rest of the population[18]. Suicide among older adults is associated with diagnosable psychopathology, most often major depression, in approximately 90% of the cases[18]. Depression can also influence decision-making capacity and may be the cause of indirect life-threatening behavior such as refusal of food, medications, or other treatments in elderly patients[19]. Studies have also shown that more than half of those over age 65 visited a physician within 1 week of death, 75% within 1 month, and 90% within 3 months[16,20,21]. Most of the patients had their first episode of major depression, which was only moderately severe, yet the depressive symptoms went unrecognized and untreated. It is in the clinical setting, therefore, that screening procedures and assessment protocols have the most direct impact.

TREATMENT FOR LATE-LIFE DEPRESSION WORKS

Depression is the most treatable of the mental disorders in late life[2]. If recognized, the treatment response for depression is good in 60% to 80% of the cases, and approximately 80% of elders can remain relapse-free with medication maintenance for 6 to 18 months[5]. Recurrence is a serious problem, with up to 40% experiencing depression chronically, especially after acute illness and hospitalization[22]. Therefore continuation treatment to prevent early relapses and longer-term maintenance treatment to prevent later recurrences is important[16]. Even in those patients with depression who have a comorbid medical illness or a dementia, treatment response is good. In patients with dementia, treatment of depression has been shown to improve cognitive performance, mood, physical and social functioning, as well as family well-being[3].

DEPRESSION IN LATE LIFE IS MISUNDERSTOOD

In spite of its prevalence, associated negative outcomes, and good treatment response, depression in older adults is highly underrecognized, misdiagnosed, and subsequently undertreated. It is estimated that as many as 90% of older adults, particularly those in institutions, who are considered to need mental health care receive no services for primary psychiatric disorders, including depression[23]. Barriers to care for older adults with depression exist at many levels. In particular, some older adults refuse to seek help because of perceived stigma of mental illness. Others may simply accept their feelings of profound sadness without realizing they are clinically depressed. Recognition of depression also is frequently obscured by anxiety, and/or the various somatic or dementia-like symptoms manifest in elderly patients with depression or because patient or providers believe that depression is a "natural" part of the aging process or is an understandable and logical reaction to medical illness, hospitalization, relocation to a nursing home, or other stressful life events. Depression—major or minor—that persists or that interferes with day-to-day functioning must not be ignored regardless of the situation or circumstances.

CAUSE AND RISK FACTORS

Several biologic and psychosocial causes for late-life depression have been proposed. Genetic factors or heredity seems to play more of a role when elders have had depression throughout their life. Additional biologic causes proposed for late-life depression include neurotransmitter or "chemical messenger" imbalance or dysregulation of endocrine function[2]. Neuroanatomic correlates, cerebrovascular disease, brain metabolism alterations, gross brain disease, and the presence of apolipoprotein E have also been etiologically linked to late-life depression[24]. Possible psychosocial causes for depression in older adults include cognitive distortions, stressful life events, especially loss, chronic stress, and low self-efficacy expectations[2,25].

The social and demographic risk factors for depression in older adults include female sex, unmarried status (particularly widowed), stressful life events, and the absence of a supportive social network[5]. In older adults there is additional emphasis on the co-occurrence of specific physical conditions such as stroke, cancer, dementia, arthritis, hip fracture surgery, myocardial infarction, chronic obstructive pulmonary disease, and Parkinson's disease. Medical comorbidity is the hallmark of depression in elderly patients and this factor represents a major difference from depression in younger populations[1]. Severe medical illness has repeatedly been shown to be among the most robust and consistent of all correlates of depression among older medical patients[14]. Those elders with functional disabilities, especially those with new functional loss, are also at risk. The more severe the medical illness and associated functional disability, the greater the likelihood of depression in elderly patients[16]. Subgroups of elderly persons who are at greater risk for major depression also include the chronically physically ill, institutionalized elders, the recently bereaved, and family members caring for the chronically ill relatives.

ASSESSMENT OF DEPRESSION IN ELDERLY PATIENTS

Table 9.1 depicts a standard of practice protocol for depression in elderly patients that emphasizes a systematic assessment guide for early recognition of depression by nurses in hospitals and other clinical settings. Early recognition of depression is enhanced by targeting high-risk groups of older adults for assessment methods that are routine, standardized, and systematic, by use of both a depression screening tool and individualized depression assessment or interview[27].

Depression Screening Tool

Nursing assessment of depression in elderly patients can be facilitated by the use of an assessment tool such as the Geriatric Depression Scale (GDS)[27]. The GDS is a 30–item self-report depression screening tool that is frequently used in a variety of clinical settings. This scale has been validated and used extensively with older adults, including those who are mentally ill, mild to moderately cognitively impaired, or institutionalized. It has a brief yes/no response format and takes approximately 10 minutes to complete. The GDS contains few somatic items that may be potentially confounded with symptoms caused by a medical illness. A GDS score of 11 or greater is considered significant for depression[27]. The GDS is not a substitute for an individualized assessment or a diagnostic interview by a mental health professional but is a useful screening tool to identify an elderly patient's depression.

Individualized Assessment and Interview

Central to the individualized depression assessment and interview is assessment of the full spectrum of symptoms (nine) for major depression as delineated by the DSM-IV[7]. Furthermore, elderly patients should be asked directly and specifically if they have been having suicidal ideation, that is, thoughts that life is not worth living or if they have been contemplating or have at-

TABLE 9.1   Nursing Standard of Practice Protocol: Depression in Elderly Patients

I. BACKGROUND

  A. Depression—Both major depressive disorders and minor depression is highly prevalent in community-dwelling, medically ill, and institutionalized elders.

  B. Depression is not a natural part of aging or a normal reaction to acute illness and hospitalization.

  C. Consequences of depression include amplification of pain and disability, delayed recovery from illness and surgery, worsening of drug side effects, excess use of health services, cognitive impairment, subnutrition, and increased suicide-and nonsuicide-related death.

  D. Depression tends to be long-lasting and recurrent. Therefore a wait-and-see approach is undesirable, and immediate clinical attention is necessary.

  E. If recognized, treatment response is good.

  F. Somatic symptoms may be more prominent than depressed mood in late life depression.

  G. Mixed depressive and anxiety features may be evident among many elderly patients.

  H. Recognition of depression is hindered by the coexistence of physical illness and social and economic problems common in late life.

  I. Early recognition, intervention, and referral by nurses can reduce the negative effects of depression.

II. ASSESSMENT PARAMETERS

  A. Identify risk factors/high risk groups.

   1. Specific physical illnesses (stroke, cancer, dementia, arthritis, hip fracture, myocardial infarction, chronic obstructive pulmonary disease, and Parkinson's disease).

   2. Functional disability (especially new functional loss).

   3. Widow/widowers.

   4. Caregivers.

   5. Social isolation/absence of social support.

  B. Assess all at-risk groups using a standardized depression screening tool and document score. The GDS is recommended because it takes approximately 10 minutes to administer, has been validated and extensively used with medically ill older adults, and includes *few* somatic items that may be confounded with physical illness.

  C. Perform an *individualized* depression assessment on all at-risk groups and document results. Note the number of symptoms; onset; frequency/patterns; duration (especially 2 weeks); change from normal mood, behavior, and functioning.

   1. Depressive symptoms

    a. Depressed or irritable mood, frequent crying.

    b. Loss of interest, pleasure (in family, friends, hobbies, sex).

    c. Weight loss or gain (especially loss)[+].

(continued)

TABLE 9.1   *(continued)*

    d. Sleep disturbance (especially insomnia)[+].
    e. Fatigue/loss of energy[+].
    f. Psychomotor slowing/agitation[+].
    g. Diminished concentration.
    h. Feelings of worthlessness/guilt.
    i. Suicidal thoughts or attempts, hopelessness.
  2. Psychosis (i.e., delusional/paranoid thoughts, hallucinations)
  3. History of depression, substance abuse (especially alcohol), previous coping style.
  4. Recent losses or crises (e.g., death of relative, friend, pet; retirement; *anniversary dates;* move to another residence, nursing home); changes in physical health status, relationships, roles.
D. Assess for depressogenic medications (e.g., narcotics, sedative/hypnotics, benzodiazepines, steroids, antihypertensives, H2 antagonists, beta-blockers, antipsychotics, immunosuppressives, cytotoxic agents, alcohol).
E. Assess for related systemic and metabolic processes (e.g., infection, anemia, hypothyroidism or hyperthyroidism, hyponatremia, hypercalcemia, hypoglycemia, congestive heart failure, kidney failure).
III. CARE PARAMETERS
A. For major depression (GDS score 11 or greater, 5 to 9 depressive symptoms [must include depressed mood or loss of pleasure] plus other positive responses on individualized assessment [especially suicidal thoughts or psychosis]), refer for psychiatric evaluation. Treatment options may include medication or cognitive-behavioral, interpersonal, or brief psychodynamic psychotherapy/counseling (individual, group, family), hospitalization, or electroconvulsive therapy.
B. For less severe depression (GDS score 11 or greater, less than five depressive symptoms plus other positive responses on individualized assessment), refer to mental health services for psychotherapy/counseling (see above types), especially for specific issues identified in individualized assessment and to determine whether medication therapy may be warranted. Consider resources such as psychiatric liaison nurses, geropsychiatric advanced practice nurses, social workers, psychologists, and other community and institution-specific mental health services. If suicidal thoughts or psychosis is present, a referral for a comprehensive psychiatric evaluation should always be made.
C. For *all* levels of depression, develop an *individualized* plan integrating the following nursing interventions
  1. Institute safety precautions for suicide risk as per institutional policy (in outpatient settings, ensure continuous surveillance of the patient while obtaining an emergency psychiatric evaluation and disposition).

(continued)

TABLE 9.1 *(continued)*

2. Remove or control etiologic agents.
   a. Avoid/remove/change depressogenic medications.
   b. Correct/treat metabolic/systemic disturbances.
3. Monitor and promote nutrition, elimination, sleep/rest patterns, physical comfort (especially pain control).
4. Enhance physical function (i.e., structure regular exercise/activity, refer to physical, occupational, recreational therapies); develop a daily activity schedule.
5. Enhance social support (i.e., identify/mobilize a support person(s) [e.g., family, confidant, friends, hospital resources, support groups, patient visitors]); ascertain need for spiritual support and contact appropriate clergy.
6. Maximize autonomy/personal control/self-efficacy (e.g., include patient in active participation in making daily schedules, short term goals).
7. Identify and reinforce strengths and capabilities.
8. Structure and encourage daily participation in relaxation therapies, pleasant activities (conduct a pleasant activity inventory).
9. Monitor and document response to medication and other therapies; readminister depression screening tool.
10. Provide practical assistance; assist with problem-solving.
11. Provide emotional support (i.e., empathic, supportive listening, encourage expression of feelings, hope instillation), support adaptive coping, encourage pleasant reminiscences.
12. Provide information about the physical illness and treatment(s) and about depression (i.e., that depression is common, treatable, and not the person's fault).
13. Educate about the importance of adherence to prescribed treatment regimen for depression (especially medication) to prevent recurrence; educate about *specific* antidepressant side effects due to personal inadequacies.
14. Ensure mental health community link-up; consider psychiatric nursing home care intervention.

IV. EVALUATION OF EXPECTED OUTCOMES
   A. Patient:
   1. Patient safety will be maintained.
   2. Patients with severe depression will be evaluated by psychiatric services.
   3. Patients will report a reduction of symptoms that are indicative of depression. A reduction in the GDS score will be evident and suicidal thoughts or psychosis will resolve.
   B. Health care provider:

(continued)

TABLE 9.1 *(continued)*

1. Early recognition of patient at risk, referral, and interventions for depression, and documentation of outcomes will be improved.
   C. Institution:
   1. The number of patients identified with depression will increase.
   2. The number of in-hospital suicide attempts will not increase.
   3. The number of referrals to mental health services will increase.
   4. The number of referrals to psychiatric nursing home care services will increase.
   5. Staff will receive ongoing education on depression recognition, assessment, and interventions.
V. FOLLOW-UP TO MONITOR CONDITION
   A. Continue to track prevalence and documentation of depression in at-risk groups.
   B. Show evidence of transfer of information to postdischarge mental-health service delivery system.
   C. Educate caregivers to continue assessment processes.

⁺Somatic symptoms, also seen in many physical illnesses, are frequently associated with no. 1 and no. 2; therefore the full range of depressive symptoms should be assessed.

From references 1, 2, 7, 9, 16, 27, 28.

tempted suicide. The number of symptoms, type, duration, frequency, and patterns of depressive symptoms, as well as a change from the patient's normal mood or functioning, would be noted. Additional components of the individualized depression assessment would include evidence of psychotic thinking, especially delusional thoughts, anniversary dates of previous losses or nodal/stressful events, previous coping style, specifically alcohol or other substance abuse, relationship changes, physical health changes, a history of depression or other psychiatric illness that required some form of treatment, a general loss and crises inventory, and any concurrent life stressors. Subsequent questioning of the family or caregiver is then recommended to obtain further information about the elder's verbal and nonverbal expressions of depression.

Differentiation of Medical or Iatrogenic Causes of Depression

Once depressive symptoms are recognized, medical and drug-related causes should be explored. Tables 9.2 and 9.3 list common

TABLE 9.2   Physical Illnesses Associated with Depression in Elderly Patients

Metabolic disturbances
    Dehydration
    Azotemia, uremia
    Acid-base disturbances
    Hypoxia
    Hyponatremia and hypernatremia
    Hypoglycemia and hyperglycemia
    Hypocalcemia and hypercalemia
Endocrine disorders
    Hypothyroidism and hyperthyroidism
    Hyperparathyroidism
    Diabetes mellitus
    Cushing's Disease
    Addison's Disease
Infections
    Viral
        Pneumonia
        Encephalitis
    Bacterial
        Pneumonia
        Urinary tract
        Meningitis
        Endocarditis
    Other
        Tuberculosis
        Brucellosis
        Fungal meningitis
        Neurosyphilis
Cardiovascular disorders
    Congestive heart failure
    Myocardial infarction, angina
Pulmonary disorders
    Chronic obstructive lung disease
    Malignancy
Gastrointestinal disorders
    Malignancy (especially pancreatic)
    Irritable bowel
    Other organic causes of chronic abdominal pain, ulcer, diverticulosis
    Hepatitis
Genitourinary disorders
    Urinary incontinence
Musculoskeletal disorders
    Degenerative arthritis

(continued)

TABLE 9.2   *(continued)*

Osteoporosis with vertebral compression or hip fractures
    Polymyalgia rheumatica
    Paget's Disease
Neurologic disorders
    Cerebrovascular disease
    Transient ischemic attacks
    Stroke
    Dementia (all types)
    Intracranial mass
        Primary or metastatic tumors
    Parkinson's disease
Other illness
    Anemia (of any cause)
    Vitamin deficiencies
    Hematologic or other systemic malignancy
Immune Disorders

---

physical illnesses and pharmacologic agents associated with depressive symptoms in elderly patients. In medically ill elderly patients, who frequently have multiple medical diagnoses and are prescribed multiple medications, these "organic" factors in the cause of depression area a major issue in nursing assessment[29]. In collaboration with the patient's physician, efforts should be directed toward treatment, correction, or stabilization of associated metabolic or systemic conditions, and, when medically feasible, depressogenic medications should be eliminated, minimized, or substituted for those that are less depressogenic.

CLINICAL DECISION MAKING AND TREATMENT

Regardless of the setting, elderly patients who exhibit the number of symptoms indicative of a major depression, specifically suicidal thoughts or psychosis, and who score *above* the established cut-off score for depression on a depression screening tool (e.g., 10 on the GDS) should be referred for a comprehensive psychiatric evaluation. Elderly patients with less severe depressive symptoms without suicidal thoughts or psychosis but who also score *above* the cut-off score on the depression screening tool (e.g., 10 on the GDS) should be referred to available psychosocial services (i.e., psychiatric liaison nurses, geropsychiatric advanced practice

TABLE 9.3   Drugs Used to Treat Physical Illness that can cause Symptoms of Depression in Elderly Patients

Antihypertensives
    Reserpine
    Methyldope
    Propranolol
    Clonidine
    Hydralazine
    Guanethidine
    Diuretics*
Analgesics
    Narcotic
    Morphine
    Codeine
    Meperidine
    Pentazocine
    Propoxphene
Nonnarcotic
    Indomethacin
Antiparkinsonian agents
    L-Dopa
Antimicrobials
    Sulfonamides
    Isoniazid
Cardiovascular agents
    Digitals
    Lidocaine+
Hypoglycemic agents++
Steroids
    Corticosteroids
    Estrogens
Others
    Cimetidine
    Cancer chemotherapeutic agents

*By causing dehydration or electrolyte imbalance.
+Toxicity.
++By causing hypoglycemia.

nurses, social workers, psychologists) for psychotherapy or other psychosocial therapies, as well as to determine whether medication for depression is warranted.

The two major categories of treatment for depression in older adults are biologic therapies (e.g., pharmacotherapy and electroconvulsive therapy) and psychosocial therapies (e.g., psychotherapies such as cognitive-behavioral, interpersona, and brief psychodynamic) in both individual and group formats[5]. Marital and family therapy may also be beneficial in treating elders with depression. The type and severity of depressive symptoms influence the type of treatment approach. In general, more severe depression, especially with suicidal thoughts or psychosis, requires intensive psychiatric treatment including hospitalization, medication with an antidepressant or antipsychotic drug, electroconvulsive therapy, and intensive psychosocial support[2]. Less severe depression without suicidal thoughts or psychosis may require treatment with psychotherapy or medication, often on an outpatient basis.

INDIVIDUALIZED NURSING INTERVENTIONS FOR DEPRESSION

Psychosocial and behavioral nursing interventions can be incorporated into the plan of care, based on the patient's individualized need. Provision of safely precautions for patients with suicidal thinking is a priority. In acute medical settings, patients may require transfer to the psychiatric service when suicidal risk is high and staffing is not adequate to provide continuous observation of the patient. In outpatient settings, continuous surveillance of the patient should be provided while an emergency psychiatric evaluation and disposition is obtained.

Promotion of nutrition, elimination, sleep/rest patterns, physical comfort, and pain control has been recommended specifically for depressed medically ill elderly patients[29]. Relaxation strategies should be offered to relieve anxiety and as an adjunct to pain management. Nursing interventions should also focus on enhancement of the elder's physical function through structured and regular activity and exercise, referral to physical, occupational and recreational therapies, and the development of a daily activity schedule; enhancement of social support by identifying, mobilizing, or designing a support person such as family, a confidant, friends, volunteers and other hospital resources, church member, support groups, patient or peer visitors, and particularly by accessing appropriate clergy for spiritual support; and maximization of the elder's autonomy, personal control, self-efficacy, and decision-making about clinical care, daily schedules, and personal routines[30]. The use of a graded task assignment where a larger goal or task is subdivided into several small steps can be helpful in enhancing function, assuring successful experiences, and building elderly patients' confidence in their performance of various activities[29]. Participation in regular, predictable, pleasant activities can result in more positive mood changes for elderly patients with depression[31]. A pleasant events inventory, elicited from the patient, can be used to incorporate pleasurable activities in to the elderly patient's daily schedule[31].

Pleasant reminiscences can enhance self-esteem and sometimes alleviate a depressed mood[32]. Nursing interventions to encourage reminiscence include asking patients directly about their past or by linking events in history with the patient's life experience. The use of photographs, old magazines, scrapbooks, and other objects can also stimulate discussion. Nurses should provide emotional support to depressed elderly patients by providing empathetic, supportive listening, encouraging patients to express their feelings in a focused manner on issues such as grief or role transition, supporting adaptive coping strategies, identifying and reinforcing strengths and capabilities, maintaining privacy and respect, and instilling hope.

Elderly patients should be closely monitored for therapeutic response and potential side effects of antidepressant medications and to assess whether dose adjustment of antidepressant medication may be warranted. Although, in general, it is necessary to start antidepressant medication at low doses in elderly patients, it is also necessary to ensure that elders with persistent depressive symptoms receive adequate treatment[33]. In particular, it is important to increase the patient's awareness of their symptoms as part of a depression that is treatable and not the person's fault as a result of personal inadequacies.

CONCLUSIONS

Depression significantly threatens the personal integrity and "experience of life" of older adults. Depression is often reversible with prompt and appropriate treatment (Box 1). Early recognition can be enhanced by the use of a standardized protocol that outlines a systematic method for depression assessment. Early identification of depressed elders and subsequent intervention and successful treatment demonstrates to society that depression is the most treatable mental problem in late life. As Blazer[8] stated "When there is depression, hope remains."

REFERENCES

[1] Lebowitz BD. Diagnosis and treatment of depression in late life an overview of the NIH consensus statement. *J Am Geriatr Soc.* 1996;4(Suppl. I):S3–S6.

[2] Blazer DG. *Depression in Late Life.* (2nd ed.) St. Louis: Mosby-Year Book; 1993.

[3] Teri L, Wagner A. Alzheimer's disease and depression. *J Consult Clin Psychol.* 1992;60:379–391.

[4] Pearson JL, Teri L, Reifler BV. Functional status and cognitive impairment in Alzheimer's patients with and without depression. *J Am Geriatr Soc.* 1989;34:1117–1121.

[5] NIH Consensus Development Panel. Diagnosis and treatment of depression in late life. *JAMA.* 1992;268:1018–1024.

[6] Blazer DG, Hughes DC, George LK. The epidemiology of depression in an elderly community population. *Gerontologist* 1987;27:281–287.

[7] American Psychiatric Association. Diagnostic and Statistical Manual of Mental Disorders. 4th ed. Washington, DC: American Psychiatric Association; 1994.

[8] Blazer DG. Depression in the elderly. *N Engl J Med.* 1989;320:164–166.

[9] Kurlowicz LH. Depression in hospitalized medically ill elders: Evolution of the concept. *Arch Psychiatr Nurs.* 1994;8:124–126.

[10] Cohen-Mansfield J, Werner P, Marx MS. Screaming in nursing home residents. *J Am Geriatr Soc.* 1990;38:785–792.

BOX 1.   Case Example

Mrs. M. is a 76-year-old woman who had depression for the first time in late life while experiencing a series of psychosoical stresses, including caring for a husband with Alzheimer's dementia and multiple physical illnesses, relocating from her lifelong home, separation from friends, major surgery and subsequent convalescence, and the eventual death of her husband. Mrs. M. was unable to function in her daily life, no longer enjoyed her pastimes, and had contemplated suicide, but never thought of herself as being depressed. Recognition of her depressive symptoms by her nurse during an acute care hospitalization, subsequent referral to the geropsychiatric consultation liaison nurse, and psychiatric visiting nurse intervention after discharge helped Mrs. M. see her symptoms as being part of a treatable depression. She agreed to a psychiatric evaluation, and antidepressant therapy was initiated. She also participated in individual psychotherapy, a bereavement support group sponsored by her church, and a senior outreach program provided through a local agency on aging. Mrs. M's therapeutic response to the various interventions was good. Her depressive symptoms diminished, she no longer contemplated suicide, and her daily physical and social functioning improved. Several months later she stated: "I'm not happy, mind you—I'm still mourning the loss of my husband of 55 years, and it's a struggle some days, but I now have hope that things will get better."

---

[11] Koenig HG, Blazer DG. Minor depression in late life. *Am J Geriatr Psych.* 1996;4(Suppl. I):S14–S21.

[12] Broadhead WE, Blazer DG, George LK, Tse CK. Depression, disability days, and days lost from work in a prospective epidemiologic survey. *JAMA.* 1990;264:2524–2528.

[13] Wells KD, Stewart A, Hays RD, Burnam A, Rogers W, Daniels M, et al. The functioning and well-being of depressed patients results from the medical outcomes study. *JAMA.* 1989;262:914–919.

[14] Koenig HG, Meador KG, Cohen HJ, Blazer DG. Depression in elderly patients with medical illness. *Arch Intern Med.* 1988;148:1929–1936.

[15] Katz IR. On the inseparability of mental and physical health in aged persons. Lessons from depression and medical comorbidity. *Am J Geriatr Psychiatr.* 1996;4:1–16.

[16] Katz IR, Streim J, Parmalee P. Prevention of depression, recurrences, and complications in late life. *Preventive Med.* 1994;23:743–750.

[17] Parmalee PA, Katz IR, Lawton MP. Depression and mortality among institutionalized elderly. *J Gerontol.* 1992;47:P3–P10.

[18] Conwell Y. Suicide in the elderly. In: Schneider LS, Reynolds BD,

Lebowitz BD, Friedhoff AJ. Eds. *Diagnosis and Treatment of Depression in Late Life: Results of the NIH Consensus Development Conference.* Washington, DC: American Psychiatric Press; 1994.

[19] Conwell Y, Caine ED, Olsen K. Suicide and cancer in late life. *Hosp Comm Psychiatr.* 1990;41:1334–1338.

[20] Barraclough BM, Bunch J, Nelson B. A hundred cases of suicide: Clinical aspects. *Br J Psychiatr.* 1974;125:355–373.

[21] Miller M. Geriatric suicide. The Arizona study. *Gerontologist.* 1978;18:488–495.

[22] Koenig HG, George L, Peterson B, Pieper C, Fowler N, Sanfelippo T. Course of depression and predictors of recovery in medically ill hospitalized elderly: A preliminary report. *Gerontol Abs.* 1996;36.

[23] Burns BJ, Taub CA. Mental health services in general medical care and in nursing homes. In: Fogel BS, Furino A, Gottlieb G, Eds. In: *Mental Health Policy for Older Americans: Protecting Minds at Risk.* Washington, DC: American Psychiatric Press; 1990.

[24] Krishnan KR, Gadde KM. The pathophysiologic basis for late life depression. *Am J Geriatr Psychiatr.* 1996;4(Supp. I):S22–S33.

[25] Holahan CK, Holahan CJ. Self-efficacy, social support, and depression in aging: A longitudinal analysis. *J Gerontol.* 1987;42:65–68.

[26] Keane SM, Sells S. Recognizing depression in the elderly. *J Gerontol Nurs.* 1990;16:21–25.

[27] Yesabage JA, Brink TL, Rose TL, Lum O, Huang V, Adey M, et al. Development and validation of a geriatric depression screening scale: a preliminary report. *J Psychiatr Res.* 1983;17:37–49.

[28] Dreyfus JK. Depression assessment and interventions with medically ill frail elderly. *J Gerontol Nurs.* 1988;14:27–36.

[29] Parmalee PA, Katz IR, Lawton MP. The relation of pain to depression among institutionalized aged. *J Gerontol.* 1991;46:15–21.

[30] Koenig HG. Depressive disorders in older medical inpatients. *Am Fam Pract.* 1991;44:1243–1250.

[31] Teri L, Logsdon RG. Identifying pleasant activities for Alzheimer's disease patients-AD. *Gerontol.* 1991;46:15–21.

[32] Osborn C. Reminiscence: when the past meets present. J Gerontol Nurs. 1989:15:6–12.

[33] American Association of Geriatric Psychiatry. Position statement. Psychotherapeutic medication in nursing homes. *J Am Geriatr Soc.* 1992;40:946–949.

Chapter 10

ENSURING MEDICATION SAFETY FOR OLDER ADULTS

Mary K. Walker, Marquis D. Foreman, and the NICHE Faculty

EDUCATIONAL OBJECTIVES:

On completion of this chapter, the reader should be able to:
1. Identify three factors that place older adults at risk for medication problems.
2. Specify four classes of medications having a high potential for toxicity in the elderly.
3. Conduct a comprehensive medication assessment.
4. Plan strategies to counteract some common drug-induced problems in older adults.
5. Develop an individualized plan to promote medication safety in an older adult.

MEDICATION SAFETY: A PROTOCOL FOR NURSING ACTION

Adults become increasingly susceptible to adverse drug effects as they age. Physiologic changes characteristic of aging predispose older adults to experience more adverse drug effects than adults under the age of 65 years. Persons over the age of 65 years experience medication problems from three major sources: (1) age-related physiologic changes that result in altered pharmacokinetics and pharmacodynamics (inability to clear and excrete medications; and alterations in blood-brain barrier integrity that predict central penetration); (2) multiple medication prescriptions (polypharmacy) to manage chronic illnesses, often written by multiple providers, and (3) medication consumption for the treatment of age-related symptoms that are not disease dependent or specific (self-medication). Susceptibility to adverse drug effects comes at a time when many elders are at risk for injury from environmental as well as therapeutic sources[1]. Although the precise physiologic and pharmacologic explanations of these adverse reactions are beyond the scope of this chapter, interested readers are referred to several chapters and articles that are useful for understanding these complex responses in elders[2,3].

Older adults represent a targeted group for medication prescription and consumption in this country[4,5]. Estimates indicate that 25% to 40% of all medication prescriptions written in the United States are for older persons[5–8]. Their susceptibility to drug-induced health problems is mirrored in estimated hospital admission rates for drug-related problems and toxicity ranging between 10% and 33%[6,9].

The average community-dwelling older adult takes between four and six medications daily and fills thirteen prescriptions annually[8]. Hospitalized adults, on the other hand, consume nine medications a day during hospitalization[10]. Further, medication treatment extends into the subacute and early discharge periods following hospitalization as well. Conn et al. found in a sample of 179 recently discharged adults aged 65–101 years that subjects were discharged from acute care facilities with a total of 950 prescriptive medications that were to be filled and properly consumed, often without patient education or oversight[9]. Thus, medications are prescribed and consumed by elders in rates and amounts that exceed that of the general population despite the fact that medications are often known to be less effective or unnecessary[5]. Such prescriptive practices predict therapeutic misadventure mirrored in admission or readmission to acute care facilities for treatment of medication-related problems.

HIGH RISK MEDICATIONS

Walker, among others[3,4,6,8,11] identified a variety of medication classes that have a relatively high potential for toxicity and adverse effects in elders. These include many commonly administered medications that are assumed, but not demonstrated, to be effective in aging persons.

Antihypertensives Agents

Hypertension affects a sizeable portion of the elderly population. It appears, however, that elderly persons are less tolerant of the potential side effects of this class of medications than their non-elderly counterparts. Of particular importance in this population is the tendency to be susceptible to the full spectrum of drug action in the presence of increased potential for injury. The antihypertensives, as a class, tend to produce a variety of unintended effects including orthostatic hypotension, sedation, depressive symptoms, impotence, and constipation[12]. These unintended effects occur even in individuals under the age of 65 years. Thus, comprehensive and ongoing assessment is key to monitoring drug efficacy.

Because of changes in fat/lean body mass that characterize the aging process, elders generally do not tolerate fat-soluble beta blockers. Indeed, dose for dose, water-soluble compounds are more potent in aging persons, whereas fat-soluble drugs can be expected to have an extended half-life. Additionally, changes in central penetration that occur as a result of age-related decreases in integrity of the blood–brain barrier predispose elders to untoward experiences with alpha agonists as well. Alterations in cognitive status, particularly confusion and dementia-like states, have been reported in elders consuming these medications for control of hypertension[13].

The angiotensin-converting enzyme inhibitors (ACE-inhibitors) are known to reduce renal function in the presence of renal clearance already compromised by aging. The net effect of such drug action is to increase the actual amount of circulating drug because older adults cannot clear the medication at the same rate as younger adults. Thus, drug toxicity can be predicted as a result of the interaction of known drug properties with physiologic effects of aging. Orthostatic hypotension is a critical problem affecting elders on sustained antihypertensive therapy. Indeed, hypovolemia is a frequent physical covariate for hypertensive persons who are orthostatic[8]. Known sequelae of orthostatic hypotension in elders include falls. Because of increased susceptibility to injury, falls represent true trauma and a medical emergency in physically frail or functionally compromised elders. Sequelae of falls, including hip fracture and head trauma, account for almost 60% of drug-related injuries and contribute to 6% of patient deaths in this population[1,14–15], notably from problems associated with immobility (e.g., pneumonia, embolus).

Psychoactive Drugs

Major psychiatric symptoms and disorders occur in 15% to 25% of persons over the age of 65 years[16]. Additionally, older persons comprise 29% of residents in state mental hospitals. Over 80% of residents in long-term care facilities experience psychiatric illnesses or exhibit behavioral alterations severe enough to be considered candidates for psychotropic drug administration. Indeed, Avorn, Dreyer, Connelly, and Soumerai documented that 39% of long-term care residents received antipsychotic drug therapy[19].

Sleep problems are frequent correlates of depressive, psychotic, or demented symptomatology in aging persons. Prevailing clinical norms aside, the use of sedative-hypnotics in elderly persons should generally be avoided at all costs. Oversedation, respiratory depression, confusion, and other alterations in cognitive capacity, as well as falls are frequent correlates of sedative-hypnotic use. Cadieux and Foreman, Wykle, and the NICHE Faculty suggest the adoption of regular sleep-wake schedules, avoiding caffeine and alcohol consumption, reducing daytime naps, and avoiding stimulant medications as measures to maximize ability to sleep[20,21].

Psychoactive medications include antidepressants (tricyclics, SSRI's), anxiolytics agents (e.g., diazepam), antipsychotics (neuroleptics), mood-stabilizing compounds (lithium), and psychoactive stimulants, in addition to the sedative-hypnotics. These latter medications are known to have relatively narrow therapeutic windows even in fully functional, nonelderly adults. Psychoactive compounds are most frequently prescribed for sedation of agitated behaviors, stabilization of mood, and pharmacotherapeutic effects in true depressive states. However, elders are at risk when consuming these medications because of changes in absorption, metabolism, distribution, and excretion of both parent drug and psychoactive metabolites. Further, these changes predict unintended interactions that require careful surveillance on the part of sensible clinicians.

Half-lives of psychoactive drugs are extended in aging persons and, in general, this class of drugs must be used with extreme caution to avoid producing falls and other traumatic injury in elders consuming these drugs. As an example, diazepam, an antianxiety agent, has a known half-life of at least 8–12 hours in adults. However, one of its major metabolites is known to have a half-life of 54 hours, even in persons whose hepatic and renal clearance is intact. Circulating levels of parent drug and metabolite are extended in persons over the age of 65 years; therefore, the dose of drug administered and the frequency of drug administration become critical considerations when medicating older adults.

Further, the risk of adverse drug effects increases exponentially with the numbers of drugs administered, as well as with the doses of drug used in therapeutic intervention. Cadieux[20] documents that when five drugs are prescribed, the potential for adverse reactions approaches 50%, whereas Sloan[22] argues that the likelihood for untoward effects is nearly 100% when 8 medications are prescribed and consumed.

Although antianxiety agents, such as the benzodiazepines and sedative-hypnotics, are generally overprescribed in elders, the antidepressants are generally considered by knowledgeable clinicians to be underprescribed. It is estimated that almost 15% of older persons living in the community have significant depressive symptoms[23]. The numbers of depressed elders increase if individuals who are institutionalized in psychiatric and long-term care facilities, as well as high-acuity environments, are added to these numbers.

A major deterrent to antidepressant pharmacotherapy in this population relates to the high incidence of anticholinergic side effects that occur with administration of these potentially beneficial psychotropic medications. Side effects such as dry mouth, blurred vision, and urinary retention, particularly in the presence of prostatic enlargement, cognitive alterations, cardiotoxicity, and constipation signal the vigilant clinician that the antidepressant profile needs to be reevaluated and likely adjusted. Tricyclic antidepressant medications with low anticholinergic profiles include desipramine, nortriptyline, and trazodone. Fluoxetine hydrochloride (Prozac) and sertraline hydrochloride (Zoloft) are relatively new nontricyclic antidepressant medications with a low incidence of anticholinergic effects. However, drug studies in elders are limited and thus, use of these medications for treatment of depressive symptoms should be judicious.

For persons over the age of 65 years presenting with agitation and behavioral problems associated with dementia, the antipsychotics are often considered firstline pharmacotherapeutic interventions[24]. Their use, however, has received increasing scientific attention. Currently, many investigators and clinicians believe that these drugs have questionable efficacy in elders. Additionally, these potent drugs must be used with extreme caution in this population, largely because of the potential for development of abnormal, and often irreversible, involuntary movements associated with administration of neuroleptics (drug-induced parkinsonism and tardive dyskinetic movements, for example). Additionally, antipsychotic drug administration is associated with a two-fold increase in potential for hip fracture from falls[25].

Anticholinergics

Drugs with high anticholinergic properties need to be used with caution in older adults for several reasons. These drugs include not only the antidepressant and neuroleptic medications previously mentioned, but medications with high anticholinergic effects including antihistamines, and intestinal and bladder relaxants[8]. In addition to their common adverse effects, administration of drugs with high anticholinergic properties is frequently associated with upper GI bleeding, particularly in older adults consuming nonsteroidal antinflammatory agents (NSAIDs) for treatment of arthritic symptoms. In those who do develop frank upper GI bleeding, the mortality rate is estimated between 10% to 20%[11]. Syncopal events and falls are common sequelae of high anticholinergic drug use, again resulting in increased morbidity and mortality in aging persons.

Cardiotonics

The current state of the science suggests that the use of digoxin for congestive heart failure in patients with normal cardiac rhythm is questionable[26,27]. A subset of patients with ventricular gallops (poor systolic ejection fractions), however, do benefit from their use. Because the therapeutic window for this drug is narrow and because it is water-soluble, dosing of older adults is a very difficult task. Digitalis toxicity in older adults is associated with visual disturbances, alterations in rate and rhythm of cardiac function, and death. Thus, current clinical thinking embraces verification of the presence and degree of systolic dysfunction prior to prescribing this potentially lethal medication[8].

Over-the-Counter Medications

Pollow et al. document that it is essential to detail the kinds and amounts of over-the-counter medications (OTCs) commonly consumed by older adults. Among these medications are analgesics, antacids, cold remedies, decongestants, fluid pills, laxatives, and herbal preparations[4]. Lamy noted that salicylates, such as aspirin, are of significant concern in explaining adverse drug reactions in older persons[28]. Additionally, cold remedies that include alcohol are a significant source of drug potentiation in aging persons. Indeed, alcohol consumption is frequently omitted from histories in elders, though it is well known that alcohol, because of its water solubility, is a potent drug that interacts with OTC and prescription medications in frank and subtle ways to produce unintended drug harm.

COMPREHENSIVE MEDICATION ASSESSMENT

Comprehensive medications assessment as suggested by Pesznecker and colleagues[29], begins with a thorough drug history and assessment obtained from the older adult or a reliable informant. Specific questions including the following:

- Ascertain the numbers and types of medications typically consumed, along with some estimate of how long the older adult has been taking the drug. It is recommended that elders collect and bring all medications to a provider to document medication types, instructions for self-administration, dates, and duration. Directed questions by the provider logically address nicotine and alcohol self-administration, as well as vitamins, herbal preparations, and over-the-counter medications that are included in the medication profile. This method allows documentation of multiple prescribing providers and dispensing pharmacies and signals of polypharmacy and/or possible substance abuse, particularly with analgesics, anxiolytics, and sedative-hypnotics.
- Query whether the elder understands what the drug is to be used for, how often it is to be taken, circumstances of ingestion (e.g., with food), and other aspects of drug self-administration that signal intelligent drug use. Ask the older adult to tell you about circumstances in which the drug has *not* been used or has been used differently than prescribed.
- Ask directly whether the elder believes that the drug is actually doing what it is intended to do. Reiterate that you are only trying to obtain accurate information, and that accurate information is the most important aspect of the interaction.
- Assess beliefs, concerns, and problems related to medication regimen. This assessment should include an evaluation of technical factors, for example, the ability to read the medica-

tion label, to open the medication container, and consume or self-administer the prescribed medication as intended.

- Discuss the impact of medication expenses. Many medications, particularly those that are newly released, are prohibitively expensive, particularly for persons on fixed incomes. Ask about concerns that the older persons may have about the costs and risks of administration. Use the opportunity to provide important information in a clear, uncomplicated manner. Provide drug sheets or other written materials when these are available, even when an individual has been using a medication for a long time.
- Ask about over-the-counter and "recreational" drug, alcohol use, and herbal or other folk remedies; be specific about the actual amount and under what circumstances these substances are used. Accurate information can help explain symptoms that otherwise may not make sense.
- Determine if PRN medications are understood. PRN medications are a mystery to many elders. Discussing the circumstances for consuming these drugs is an important aspect of patient education that promotes safe drug use.
- Assess for sensory or functional impairments and the devices used to remedy such sensory alterations. For example, tamper-proof lids are often difficult for elders to remove, particularly if they are experiencing arthritic changes. A simple request to the pharmacist to provide a nonchildproof lid may improve the safe and effective use of prescribed medication.
- Assess cognitive, and affective status to assure that memory problems or vegetative symptoms associated with depression are not interfering with the safe use of prescription drugs (see chapter 5 in this book)[30].
- Specifically ask about the circumstances of medication storage and other aspects, such as how drugs are dispensed daily, that signal a true understanding of these aspects of medication safety.
- Consider instrumental issues related to drug use, such as availability of family members or other social supports to facilitate medication compliance, how prescriptions are actually filled and reimbursed, and who monitors medication changes dictated by third-party reimbursement.

SUMMARY AND CONCLUSIONS

Medication safety is a major concern in the elderly. Although intending to remedy the signs and symptoms of disease and illness, drug misadventures are all too frequently encountered. To ensure therapeutic effects of pharmacotherapy, we have developed the accompanying guidelines such as the protocol of medication safety, which addresses the: (1) knowledge and skill necessary for performance of a medication assessment, (2) accurate and comprehensive documentation of the assessment, and (3) development of an individualized plan to promote medication safety in older adults (see Table 10.1, pp. 142–144).

REFERENCES

[1] Tinetti ME, Speechley M, Ginter SF. Risk factors for falls among elderly persons living in the community. *N Engl J Med.* 1988;319:1701–1707.
[2] Schwertz DW, Buschmann MBT. Pharmacogeriatrics. *Crit Care Nurs Q.* 1989;12(1):26–37.
[3] Walker MK. Drugs and the critically ill older adult. In TT. Fulmer & MK. Walker (Eds.), *Critical care nursing of the elderly.* New York: Springer Publishing Co. 1992:83–101.
[4] Pollow R, Stoller E, Forster L, Duniho T. Drug combinations and potential for risk of adverse drug reaction among community-dwelling elderly. *Nurs Res.* 1994;43(1):44–49.
[5] Tideiksaar R. Principles of drug therapy in the elderly. *Phys Assist.* 1990;20:29–52.
[6] DeMaagd G. High-risk drugs in the elderly population. *Geriatr Nurs.* 1995;16:198–207.
[7] Falvo D, Holland B, Brenner J, Benshoff J. Medication use practices in the ambulatory elderly. *Health Val.* 1990;3(14):10–16.
[8] Hobson, M. Medications in older patients. *West J Med.* 1992;157:539–543.
[9] Conn V, Taylor S, Steinmann A. Medication management by recently hospitalized older adults. *J Commun Health Nurs.* 1992;9(1):1–11.
[10] Montamat SC, Cusack B. Overcoming problems with polypharmacy and drug misuse in the elderly. *Clin Geriatr Med.* 1992;8(1):143–158.
[11] Katz, M. Anticholinergic increase of adverse drug reactions in elderly. *Provider.* 1993;20:53–62.
[12] Applegate WB, Miller ST. Choice of antihypertensive medication regimen. *Clin Geriatr Med.* 1989;5(4):803–811.

[13] Applegate WB, Rutan GH. Advances in management of hypertension in older persons. *J Am Geriatr Soc.* 1992;40(11):1164–1174.

[14] Rebenson-Piano M. The physiologic changes that occur with aging. *Crit Care Nurs Qu.* 1998;12(1):1–14.

[15] Tinetti ME, Speechley M. Prevention of falls among the elderly. *New Engl J Med.* 1989;320:1055–1059.

[16] Wanich CK, Sullivan-Marx EM, Gottlieb GL, Johnson JC. Functional status outcomes of a nursing intervention in hospitalized elderly. *Image: J Nurs Scholar.* 1995;24:201–207.

[17] Cadieux R, Kales, Zimmerman. *Am Fam Phys.* 1985;131(5):105–111.

[18] Rovner BW, Steele CD, German P, Clark R, Folstein MF. Psychiatric diagnosis and uncooperative behavior in nursing homes. *J Geriatr Psychia Neurol.* 1992;5:102–105.

[19] Avorn J, Dreyer P, Connelly K, Soumerai SB. Use of psychotropic medication and the quality of care in rest homes. *N Engl J Med.* 1989;320:227–232.

[20] Cadieux R. Geriatric psychopharmacology: A primary care challenge. *Postgrad Med.* 1993;4(93):281–301.

[21] Foreman MD, Wykle M, the NICHE Faculty. Nursing standard of practice protocol: sleep disturbances in elderly patients. *Geriatr Nurs.* 1995;16:238–43.

[22] Sloan RW. Drug interactions. *Am Fam Physic.* 1985;27(2):229–238.

[23] Martin L. Day care for the elderly mentally ill. *Nurs Times.* 1990;86(23):36–37.

[24] Class CA, Schneider L, Farlow MR. Optimal management of behavioral disorders associated with dementia. *Drugs Aging.* 1997;10:95–106.

[25] Ray WA, Griffin MR, Schaffner W, Baugh DK, Melton LJ III. Psychotropic drug use and the risk of hip fracture. *N Engl J Med.* 1987;316:363–369.

[26] Luchi RJ, Taffet GE, Teasdale TA. Congestive heart failure in the elderly. *J Am Geriatr Soc.* 1991;39:810–825.

[27] Mulrow CD, Feussner JR, Velez R. Reevaluation of digitalis efficacy: New light on an old leaf. *Ann Inter Med.* 1984;101(1):113–117.

[28] Lamy P. *Prescribing for the elderly.* Littleton, MA: John-Wright. 1980.

[29] Pesznecker B, Patsdaughter C, Moody K, Albert M. Medication regimens and the home care client: A challenge for health care providers. In O'Connor K. (Ed.), *Facilitating self care practices in the elderly.* Binghamton, NY: Haworth, 1990:9–68.

[30] Foreman MD, Fletcher K, Mion LC, Simon L, the NICHE Faculty. Assessing cognitive function. *Geriatr Nurs.* 1996;17(5):228–233.

TABLE 10.1   Medication Safety: A Protocol for Nursing Action

I. BACKGROUND
  A. Definitions:
    1. Medication-related problems: Encompass unintended drug effects, adverse drug reactions, polypharmacy, drug misuse, and drug abuse.
    2. Unintended drug effect: features of drug administration that are known (e.g. orhostatic hypotension) but are not intended in the prescription or administration of the drug.
    3. Adverse drug reaction: Any noxious or unintended response to a medication.
    4. Polypharmacy: The prescription, administration, or use of more medications than are clinically indicated in a given individual.
    5. Drug misuse: The inappropriate use of a substance intended for therapeutic purposes.
    6. Drug abuse: The nontherapeutic use of any psychoactive substance that in some way adversely affects the user's life.
  B. Epidemiology:
    1. 25%-40% of all medication prescriptions written in the U.S. are for older persons (13% of U.S. population).
    2. 10%-33% of admissions to acute care hospitals are for medication related problems.
    3. Average community dwelling elders consume 4–6 medications daily.
    4. 40–50% of all over-the-counter medications are consumed by elderly persons.
    5. Hospitalized adults consume on average 9 medications daily.
  C. Sources of medication-related problems
    1. Age-related physiologic changes altering pharmacodynamics and pharmacokinetics.
    2. Multiple medication prescriptions (polypharmacy).
    3. Medication consumption for age-related symptoms (self-medication).
  D. Consequences of medication-related problems:
    1. Hospitalization.
    2. Additional physical, cognitive, and affective symptoms.
    3. Increased morbidity and mortality.
    4. Loss of functional independence.
II. HIGH RISK MEDICATIONS
  A. Antihypertensive agents:
    1. Angiotensin-converting enzyme (ACE)-inhibitors, e.g., captopril.
    2. Central alpha-agonists, e.g., clonidine, guanabenz, guanfacine, and methyldopa.
    3. Beta-blockers, e.g., propanadol.
  B. Psychoactive drugs:
    1. Antipsychotic/neuroleptic drugs, e.g., haloperidol, phenothiazines.

(continued)

TABLE 10.1 *(continued)*

    2. Sedative-hypnotics medication, e.g., chloral hydrate, benzodiazepines.
    3. Antidepressant medications, e.g., amitriptyline, doxepin.
    4. Anxiolytic medications, e.g., meprobamate.
  C. Anticholinergic drugs:
    1. Atropine, scopolamine, hyoscyamine, oxybutinin.
    2. Phenothiazines.
  D. Cardiotonics:
    1. Digoxin.
    2. Quinidine preparations.
  E. Over-the-counter medications:
    1. Analgesics.
    2. Cold and flu remedies.
    3. Nonsteroidal antiinflammatory drugs (NSAIDs).
    4. Antacids.
    5. Laxatives.
  F. H_2 receptor antagonists:
    1. Cimetidine.
    2. Rantidine.
    3. Nizatidine.
    4. Famotidine.
  G. Alcohol
  H. Folk, herbal, or other home remedies
III. NURSING ACTIONS
  A. Comprehensive Medication Assessment includes:
    1. Sources of information:
      a. Elderly individual.
      b. Family or significant others.
      c. Primary care providers.
      d. Pharmacist.
      e. Home health or visiting nurse.
      f. Review of all current medication bottles.
    2. Assessment parameters:
      a. Medical diagnoses, diseases, or health problems.
      b. History of previous adverse drug reaction(s).
      c. Numbers and types of medications.
      d. Length of time taking medication.
      e. Last time the prescription was reevaluated by a competent health care provider.
      f. Instructions for administration of medication.
      g. Deviations from prescription.
      h. Storage of medications.
      i. Intended effect(s) of medication.
      j. Adverse effect(s) of medications.

(continued)

TABLE 10.1 *(continued)*

   k. Functional, sensory, cognitive, affective, and nutritional status.
   l. Technical problems with medication use, e.g., abilty to open
      bottles and to read medication labels.
   m. Allergies.
   B. Drug Safety:
      1. Educate patients and/or significant other about:
         a. Medication regimen.
         b. Medications that interact with other medications, foods, and
            alcohol.
         c. Habit-forming and addictive medications.
         d. Methods for keeping track of medications.
         e. Signals of medication problems.
IV. EVALUATION OF EXPECTED OUTCOMES
    A. Patients will:
       1. Experience fewer medication-related problems.
       2. Understand their medication regimens.
    B. Health care providers:
       1. Will become competent in comprehensive medication assessment.
       2. Document ongoing comprehensive medication assessment.
       3. Increase their knowledge about medication safety in the elderly.
    C. Institutions will find:
       1. Decreased morbidity and mortality due to medication-related
          problems.
       2. Improved documentation of medication usage.
       3. Referral to appropriate advanced practitioners (e.g., geriatrician,
          geriatric/gerontological or psychiatric clinical nurse specialist or
          nurse practitioner, or consultation-liaison service) may increase.
V. FOLLOW-UP TO MONITOR PROTOCOL EFFECTIVENESS
    A. Staff competence in the assessment of medication use.
    B. Consistent and appropriate documentation of medication assessment.
    C. Consistent and appropriate care and follow-up in presence of a
       medication-related problems.
    D. Nature and origins of medication-related problems sought in a
       timely manner.
    E. Incidence of medication-related problems decreases.
    F. Multiple episodes of teaching and reinforcement to assure
       understanding and follow-through with appropriate medication
       administration.

From Hazzard W et al. *Principles of Geriatric Medicine & Gerontology* (3rd ed.), pp. 324,
326, 1994, McGraw-Hill Companies, New York. © 1994. With permission of The McGraw-
Hill Companies.

Chapter 11

PAIN MANAGEMENT

Terry T. Fulmer, Lorraine C. Mion, Melissa M. Bottrell, and the NICHE Faculty

EDUCATIONAL OBJECTIVES:

On completion of this chapter, the reader should be able to:
1. Discuss common misperceptions related to pain management in elders.
2. Describe the gate control theory of pain.
3. Anticipate and explain to patients common fears related to pain medication.

Pain management for the elderly person is complex, challenging, but ultimately rewarding for the nurse who learns the core knowledge for assisting the older individual who is in pain. This chapter summarizes the pain literature as it relates to elders and provides a care protocol for acute care nursing. The latter is meant as a guide for those in practice who are challenged by difficult pain-management problems and want guidelines from which to then individualize pain management care plans for the elder in need.

Reproduced from Fulmer, TT, Mion, LC, Bottrell, MM, Pain management protocol. *Geriatric Nursing*, 1996, *17*, 222–227. With permission from Mosby-Year Book, Inc.

BACKGROUND

The pain-management literature has only recently specifically addressed the elder client[1–3]. Pain management for elders is fraught with clinical questions: How much medication dosing is enough while still within the safe range? For whom and under what circumstances should the various modalities of pain relief be used? How can the nurse adequately assess pain and subsequent relief in the elderly patient with cognitive impairment? Should pain medications be given judiciously to the elderly patient or provided regularly to avoid any lapse in coverage?

Although these questions are important for all patients, they are critical questions for elderly patients because of the special issues relevant to pain management in this population. The prevalence of pain in elders is known to be twice that of younger individuals; in community-residing elders, the prevalence of pain ranges from 25% to 50%[1–4]. In long-term care settings, the prevalence of pain can be as high as 85%[1]. An alarming number of elderly patients suffer from conditions that serve as a source of chronic pain, such as arthritis, gout, and peripheral vascular disease. Furthermore, the comorbidity of illnesses in older age increases the likelihood that pain management will be a serious problem for some elders. It is evident from the limited body of literature that there has been a lack of attention to this important issue. The AHCPR[5] guidelines, although excellent and long needed in the clinical setting, do not provide the specific focus on aging that can guide those working with elders who require pain relief.

What Makes Pain Management for Elders Different?

It is important to state from the outset that a majority of general theories regarding pain and its genesis do apply to elders[6]. For example, the gate control theory, which describes pain-inhibiting potential at the spinal level[7,8], has been used to describe the mechanism of pain in all ages. The two types of pain that have been described include fast-track and slow-track pain. Symptoms for fast-track pain are described as acute, sharp, stabbing, and piercing pain. Slow-track pain is throbbing, dull, aching pain. These distinctly different types of pain are common in elders. Pain intervention strategies such as relaxation therapy[9], transcutaneous electrical nerve stimulation, and antidepressant therapy may be used less frequently with elders as a result of concern related to cognitive function, tolerance for such therapy, and lack of experience in using available therapy with the elderly population. Finally, the effect of pain on activities of daily living in elders is more pronounced than for younger individuals, which can, in turn, effect the elder's quality of life. Prevention and early intervention can prevent the downward spiral that can ensue once pain begins.

Ageist Attitudes Prevail

Common perceptions—often taken as truth—of the pain experience of elders—include the following: "All old people complain of pain," "Old people can't cooperate with complex therapies," "They can't cope with patient-administered analgesia," and "They are unreliable historians and pain reporters." Much of what we know regarding pain management has come from the cancer literature[10], which has been helpful, but more is needed with specific reference to elders. The void in scientific knowledge regarding pain and its management for elders is truly significant.

ASSESSMENT APPROACHES

Essential to pain management is a systematic approach to assessment, detection, and early intervention. Elderly individuals may underreport pain. They expect pain as a sequela of normal aging and may not bring pain to the attention of clinicians simply because they are afraid of being labeled as bothersome, hypochodriachal, or addicted. Also, the pain they live with may become second nature to their existence, and they then forget to mention it during a work-up for some other more "pressing problem," such as acute chest pain. Although no one would argue that chronic pain takes priority over acute pain, careful assessment of chronic pain needs to be an ongoing part of the health evaluation.

Several excellent pain assessment protocols are available that range in type from intensity scales to complex protocols[11]. In the hospital setting, nurses can have a significant effect on the way that pain is assessed and managed if they use a structured instrument and work continuously with the interdisciplinary team. Pain assessment and management in the acute care setting are a 24-hour-a-day process. Careful surveillance can determine the cause of the pain and the relief strategies most effective for that particular person. The team must include the older patient, who is often the best source of accurate information on how pain can be relieved. For older hospitalized patients transferred from the long-term care setting or home care system, care plans already used in those agencies should be reviewed and followed as appropriate. All nurses can relate to the scenario of the patient, newly admitted to the hospital, who has two or three agonizing days, only to later learn that the nursing assistants knew the "magic bullet" that worked at home but never discussed it because they were not asked.

MEDICATIONS

Acute pain should be treated immediately. As with any age group, elders will do poorly if left to cope with severe pain for a long period of time. Review of current or recent pain-management strategies with input from the elder, family, and community caregivers will speed the therapeutic process. Previously successful medication regimens are excellent models to begin with if not contraindicated for some specific illness. Analgesics are the most frequent first intervention for acute pain, which include nonnarcotic and narcotic analgesics. Nonnarcotics include acetaminophen-based medications and nonsteroidal antiinflammatory medications. Narcotics are categorized as agonists or antagonists of central nervous system opiate receptors and include medications such as morphine, meperide (Demerol), hydromophone (Dilaudid), and codeine. Table 11.1 lists commonly used pain medications for elders[12].

TABLE 11.1   Analgesics Commonly Used Orally for Mild to Moderate Pain

Drug	Equianalgesic dose mg*	Starting oral dose range, mg†	Comments
Nonnarcotics			
Aspirin	650	650	Often used in combination with opioid-type analgesics; antiplatelet aggregation effects
Acetaminophen	650	650	Minimal antiinflammatory properties
Ibuprofen	ND	200–400	Higher analgesic potential than aspirin
Fenoprofen	--	200–400	Similar to ibuprofen
Diflunisal (Dolobid)	ND	500–1000	Longer duration of action than ibuprofen; higher analgesic potential than asprin
Naproxen	ND	250–500	Like diflunisal
Ketorolac	ND	30–60	Higher analgesic potential than aspirin
Morphine-like agonists			
Codeine	32–65	32–65	" Weak" morphine; often used in combination with nonopioid analgesics biotransformed in part, to morphine
Oxycodone	5	5–10	Oxycodone: shorter-acting and also used in combination with nonopioid analgesics (percodan, percocet) which limits dose escalation
Meperidine	50	50–100	Shorter-acting biotransformed to normeperidine a toxic metabolite
Propoxyphene HCL	65–130	65–130	"Weak" opioid, often used in combination with nonopiod analgesics; long half-life

(continued)

TABLE 11.1   (continued)

Drug	Equianalgesic dose mg*	Starting oral dose range, mgt	Comments
Propoxyphene napsylate	50	50–100	biotransformed to potentially toxic metabolite (nonpropoxyphene)
Mixed agonist-antagonist			
Pentazocine			In combination with nonopioid; in combination with naloxone to discourage parental abuse, causes psychotomimetic effects

ND, Not determined.
* For these equianalgesic doses (see comments), the time of peak analgesia ranges from
   1.5 to 2 hours and the duration from 4 to 6 hours. Oxycodone and meperidine are
   shorter-acting (3 to 5 hrs) and diflunisal and naproxen are longer acting (8 to 12 hrs).
t These are recommended starting doses from which the optimal dose for each patient is
   determined by titration and the maximal dose limited by adverse effects.
Note. From Foley KM. *Pain management in the elderly.* In Hazzard WR, Bierman EL, Blass
JP, Effinger JR WH, Halter JB, Eds. *Principles of Geriatric Medicine.* New York: McGraw-
Hill. 1994; 000. Copyright 1994 by McGraw-Hill. Reproduced with permission.

The dose and route of pain medications are two key considerations for elders. Regulation of opiates is more difficult in elderly persons, given the age-related changes in absorption, metabolism, distribution, and excretion. Absorption time may increase or decrease, depending on what other illnesses and other medications are already present. For example, mouth breathing increases with aging, which gives rise to dry, cracked oral mucosa and a decrease in saliva available to mix with oral medications, and thus decreases the ability of the elder to swallow the pill. Lemon-glycerin swabs, although often appropriate in younger individuals, may actually increase drying of the mouth and prove to be painful in mouths that may already have sores from ill-fitting dentures or other dental appliances. Pills may actually become lodged in ill fitting dentures and may incorrectly recorded as "taken."

Injections may also prove to be unreliable, if the elder's circulation is very poor, and muscle wasting slows absorption and distribution. Rectal administration may be a viable, acceptable alternative for some medications. Morphine is available in this form. As with any medication, judicious dosing, with attention to weight, interactions with other multiple medications, allergies, and any history of adverse drug reactions is essential.

Taking pain medication may be frightening to the older patient. Fear of how they will "act" while under the influence of such medications, and worry about addiction are commonplace. Nurses can help by anticipating these feelings, sharing scenarios from past experiences with other patients, and providing the elder with as much information as they need to decide the dose and evaluation points. Pain also leaves all people feeling "out of control," with such symptoms as frustration, despair, and loss of confidence in care. Whatever can be done to enhance control can be an important pain reduction strategy in and of itself. Elders with cognitive impairment have no less feelings of loss of control and should be given the same opportunities to regain a sense of control.

The many noninvasive strategies are most appropriate to the elder who is not in a pain crisis. Once the pain crisis associated with acute, new, frightening pain has subsided, alternative therapies such as relaxation, herbal medicines, therapeutic touch and biofeedback may be explored (Box 1). Pain may be relieved by more careful attention to other factors such as caloric intake, dietary preferences, quality of the elder's sleep, and emotional well-being. An elder may be nutritionally depleted, and unable to muster the energy required to participate in a pain-management plan. Similarly, a sleep-deprived elder is unlikely to get the benefit of a pain-reduction protocol until the basic need for sleep has been met. These noninvasive means may be more valuable within a care plan that addresses the "whole" person.

SUMMARY

Inappropriate pain management leaves both the elder and the nurse feeling unfulfilled and unhappy with the care. Providing guidelines through protocols (Box 2) which can then be individu-

BOX 1.   Alternative Practices in Pain Management[13]
Culture often influences the older adult's choice of interventions for dealing with pain. The following is an illustrative, but not exhaustive, list of alternative or complementary practices sometimes used by clients from culturally diverse backgrounds for pain management. • Herbal remedies • Meditation • Progressive relaxation • Hypnosis • Yoga • Imagery • Therapeutic touch • Acupuncture or acupressure • Application of heat or cold • Music • Humor

alized with the elder and the interdisciplinary team is a rewarding approach welcomed by patients and nurses alike.

REFERENCES

[1] Ferrell BA. Pain management in elderly people. *J Am Geriatr Soc.* 1991;39:64–73.

[2] Sengstaken EA, King SA. The problems of pain and its detection among geriatric nursing home residents. *J Am Geriatr Soc.* 1993;41:541–544.

[3] McGuire L, Graffam S. Pain in the elderly. In: Stanley M, Gauntlett Beare P. (Eds.) *Gerontological nursing.* Philadelphia: F.A. Davis; 1995:297–310.

[4] Crook J, Rideout E, Browne G. The prevalence of pain complaints in a general population. *Pain.* 1984;18:299–314.

[5] Agency for Health Care Policy and Research. *Clinical Practice Guideline for Acute Pain Management: Operative or Medical Procedures and Trauma.* Washington, D.C.: US Government Printing Office, USDHHS; Feb. 1992.

[6] Pascro CL, Reed B, McCaffery M. How aging affects pain management. *Am J Nurs.* 198;98(6):12–13.

[7] Melzack R, Bromage PR. Experimental phantom limbs. *Exp Neurol.* 1974;39:261–269.

[8] Melzack R. Phantom limbs and the concept of a neuromatrix. *Trends Neurosci.* 1990;13:88–92.

[9] Benson H. *The relaxation response.* New York: Morrow; 1976.

[10] Bernabei R, Gambassi G, Lapane K, Landi F, Gatsonis C, Dunlop R, Lipsitz L, Steel K, Mor V. Management of pain in elderly patients with cancer. Sage Study Group. Systematic Assessment of Geriatric Drug Use via Epidemiology. *JAMA.* 1998;279:1877–1882.

[11] Wallace M. Assessment and management of pain in the elderly. *Med Surg Nurs.* 3(4): 293–298.

[12] Foley KM. Pain management in the elderly. In Hazzard WR, Bierman EL, Blass JP, Ettinger Jr. WH, Halter JB, Eds. *Principles of Geriatric Medicine.* New York: McGraw-Hill, 1994:317–331.

[13] Lueckenotte AG. *Gerontologic Nursing.* St. Louis: Mosby-Year Book; 1996:317.

BOX 2. Standard of Practice Protocol: PAIN Management for Hospitalized Elders

---

Standard: For all elderly patients to be pain free or at a level of pain/ discomfort acceptable to that patient.

Overview: Pain is a subjective experience which is highly prevalent in the elderly. Of particular concern are those elderly patients who have delirium or dementia, and lack advocates to help them obtain pain relief. Even in the absence of cognitive impairment, an older person's pain may be minimized, underreported, undertreated, or untreated. Fear of adverse drug reactions and side effects can inhibit a nurse's willingness to administer the medication or therapy for pain relief in the elderly. The nurse, in partnership with the interdisciplinary team that includes the patient and their significant others, is in a position to develop a care plan for optimal pain management.

I. BACKGROUND
    A. Epidemiologic pattern—Prevalence: Pain, defined as an unpleasant sensory and emotional experience arising from actual or potential tissue damage, is a common, almost universal, experience among hospitalized elders. Studies suggest pain is present in 20 to 50% of community-dwelling elders, 71% of institutionalized elders, and 83% of day hospital residents.
        1. Prevalence of pain in those 60 years of age and older is twice that of younger individuals.
        2. More than 80% of elderly persons suffer from chronic conditions, such as arthritis and peripheral vascular disease.
        3. Multiple coexisting illnesses give rise to multiple sources of pain.
    B. Elders typically have insufficient pain management.
        1. Patient-specific reasons:
            a. Cognitive impairments, such as dementia or delirium, are estimated to affect at least half of the patient's ability to report the pain.
            b. Sensory impairments, such as vision or hearing, make it difficult for clinicians to use pain assessment scales.
            c. Cultural or cohort responses to pain have been reported, such as stoic refusal to take narcotics because of stigma or fear of addiction.
            d. Because of aging changes, elders often have atypical presentations of acute pain.
        2. Clinician-specific reasons:
            a. Mistaken belief that increasing age provides increasing threshold for pain.

(continued)

BOX 2. *(continued)*

      b. Lack of knowledge regarding multiple sources of pain.

      c. Misunderstanding or lack of knowledge regarding pain-medication management.

      d. Lack of agreement on assessing and interpreting elder's presentation of pain.

C. Because of the multiple disease conditions present in elders, the clinician must assess and treat elderly for two types of pain conditions:

    1. Chronic pain, defined as having a duration of 3 months or longer, has no autonomic signs (e.g., tachycardia), is usually out of proportion and not indicative of danger and is associated with long-standing functional and psychological impairment. This type of pain requires a multidimensional approach of nonpharmacologic strategies, as well as analgesics.

    2. Acute pain implies the existence of endangering injury and remedial disease. It is usually associated with autonomic activity (tachycardia, diaphoresis, mild hypertension). Control of pain relies initially on treatment of underlying condition and short-term administration of analgesic drugs.

D. Outcomes—If left unmanaged or inappropriately controlled, pain in elders is associated with the following:

    1. Depression and decreased socialization.

    2. Diminished function and ability to maintain independence while performing activities of daily living.

    3. Exacerbation of cognitive impairment.

    4. Sleep disturbance.

    5. Increased health care utilization and costs.

II. ASSESSMENT PARAMETERS

Assumptions: More than 80% of hospitalized elderly patients suffer acute and/or chronic pain conditions with known adverse consequences for function and quality of life, a routine and comprehensive assessment is necessary for each elderly patient. Assessment then must be frequent and ongoing to assess effectiveness of therapy.

A. At baseline include patient's perceptions and typical responses; it is useful to gather information from family members. Focus on verbal, nonverbal/behavioral expressions, and functional status. Assess the following:

    1. What pain-control methods have previously been helpful.

    2. Attitude toward use of opioid, anxiolytic, other substances.

    3. Function, such as gait, transfers.

    4. Depressive mood or presence of cognitive impairments.

B. Pain characteristics; various tools are available to assess the following:

(continued)

BOX 2. *(continued)*

---

1. Location.
2. Intensity.
3. Frequency.
4. Onset and duration.
5. Quality.
6. Manner of expressing pain.
C. Frequent and ongoing evaluation necessary to assess effectiveness of pain management is necessary. Elderly may have difficulty using 10–point visual analogue scale. Use of 4–point numerical scale with Pain Affect Faces Scale has been shown to be quick and reliable with elders.
D. Assess routinely for adverse effects from medications giving rise to more discomfort: e.g., urinary retention with PCA pumps, gastric ulceration with NSAIDs.
III. CARE STRATEGIES
A. Ongoing assessment of therapeutic effectiveness at baseline and throughout hospital stay is essential for all pain control strategies. The best assessment technique is patient's self-report.
B. Prevention: anticipating and instituting aggressive treatment for pain before, during and after all painful diagnostic and/or therapeutic procedures is essential to optimize both short-term and long-term outcomes. Objective is to keep patients pain-free or within acceptable limits. Strategies include:
   1. Educational strategies for patients and clinicians to utilize prophylactic medications prior to and after painful procedures.
   2. Educational strategies for patients on non-pharmacologic behavioral strategies, e.g., relaxation strategies.
   3. Strategies to prevent age-related conditions that lead or contribute to pain: pressure ulcers, urinary retention, fecal impaction, undernutrition.
C. Treatment guidelines: To target all sources of pain most likely require more than one pain management strategy.
   1. Pharmacologic:
      a. Elders are at increased risk for adverse drug reactions
      b. Increase surveillance and assessment because of risk of under- or over-medicating elders as well as adverse drug reactions.
      c. Maintain drug at therapeutic levels, avoid PRNs.
      d. Maintain continuity across shifts.
   2. Nonpharmacologic: Variety of techniques available and may benefit different subgroups of patients. Use of these may require specialized training and consultation with other health care professionals.

(continued)

BOX 2. *(continued)*

    a. Cognitive-behavioral techniques focus on changing the patient's perception of pain, alter pain behavior, or provide patient with greater control. Patients who are delirious or demented may not be appropriate. Examples: distraction (radio, TV, reading), education/instruction, relaxation, imagery, biofeedback.

    b. Physical agents focus on providing comfort or altering physiologic responses. Examples include heat or cold therapy and TENS units.

IV. EVALUATION OF EXPECTED OUTCOMES

  A. Patient:

    1. At discharge, the patient is pain free or at a level judged acceptable.

    2. Patient maintains functional ability to manage self-care.

    3. No iatrogenic outcomes, e.g., falls, charged cognitive state, GI upset/bleeding.

  B. Nurse:

    1. Evidence of ongoing and comprehensive pain assessment.

    2. Evidence of prompt interventional strategies.

    3. Increased knowledge regarding pain management in elderly: medication effects, assessment of pain in cognitively impaired, nonverbal, etc.

  C. Institution:

    1. Documentation of assessment, plan, and effectiveness.

    2. Referrals to specialists may increase (e.g., psychiatry, biofeedback, PT.).

    3. Referrals to outside providers may increase (e.g., pain centers).

    4. Variance from coordinated care tracks or pathways is not due to pain.

P.C.A.-patient controlled analgesic; NSAID-nonsteroidal antiinflammatory drug; PRN-as needed drug order; GI-gastrointestinal; PT-physical therapy.

Chapter **12**

USE OF PHYSICAL RESTRAINTS IN THE HOSPITAL SETTING

Lorraine C. Mion, Neville Strumpf, and the NICHE Faculty

EDUCATIONAL OBJECTIVES:

On completion of this chapter, the reader should be able to:
1. Identify the common patient risk factors for physical restraint.
2. Describe the perceived benefits of physical restraints.
3. Discuss the physical and psychologic risks as a direct or indirect result of physical restraint.
4. Identify the most common reasons nurses cite for use of physical restraints.
5. Plan nonrestraint strategies for dealing with common patient problems: falls, disruption of therapy, and agitation/confusion.

The use of physical restraints as sound clinical practice has been questioned and restricted in long-term-care settings. Although it is often the case that changes and advances in practice originate in acute care settings and flow to long-term care settings, the

Reproduced from Mion, LC, Strumpf, N, Use of physical restraints in the hospital setting: Implications for the nurse. *Geriatric Nursing*, 1994, *15*, 127–131. With permission from Mosby-Year Book, Inc.

opposite has occurred concerning restraints. Following the ground-breaking legislation of the Omnibus Reconciliation Act of 1987, the Joint Commission on Accreditation of Hospitals (JCAHO) recently provided guidelines restricting the use of physical re-straints[1,2]. The purpose of this chapter is to familiarize the reader with an overview of physical restraint use in the general hospital setting, decision making concerning restraints, and alternative methods of care for common patient care problems.

BACKGROUND

Prevalence

Although studies have shown significant decreases in the use of restraints in chronic care settings, restraints continue to be used in acute care settings[3]. Of adult patients of all ages on general hospital units, 6% to 17% are restrained[4–7]. With increasing age, the application of restraint becomes even more common; preva-lence increases to 18% to 20% among those 65 years or older, and up to 22% for those 75 years or older[4,7–9]. In other words, one out of five elderly patients on a general medical or surgical unit is restrained at some point during hospitalization.

Risk Factors

Several studies have compared restrained to nonrestrained pa-tients to determine risk factors for physical restraint. Risk for physical restraint is three to four times greater if a patient has at least one of the following characteristics: has a greater severity of illness, cognitive impairment, physical impairment, or a psychi-atric condition, has undergone a surgical procedure, or medical devices are restricting mobility (e.g., intravenous line)[6, 7]. In these studies the age of the patient was not a significant factor. Thus, regardless of age, hospitalized patients who exhibit confu-sion, poor judgement, or behavioral problems combined with physical impairments are those most likely to be restrained.

Benefits

Physical restraints have been defended on the grounds that they protect the patient from harm, especially harm that could occur from falling. If physical restraints were truly beneficial and effective, one would expect that no falls would occur with the use of physical restraints and that falls would increase without the use of physical restraints. Studies have shown, however, that 13% to 47% of older patients who fall are physically restrained and that serious injuries from falls are greater with the presence of physical restraints[10–16]. Although no clinical trials have tested the effectiveness of physical restraints as an intervention to prevent falls, Powell et al.[17] demonstrated no increase in fall-related injuries 4 years after implementing a restraint-reduction program in a hospital setting. Therefore it is reasonable to conclude that use of physical restraints to prevent falls is questionable.

Physical restraints have also been used to prevent disruption of therapy. A recent study revealed that physical restraint did not necessarily prevent extubation. As with the perception that physical restraint prevents injuries from falls, the use of physical restraints to promote or maintain medical treatments may also be a matter of perceived benefit.

Risks

There have been numerous reports on the risks that occur, either directly or indirectly, as a result of the use of physical restraints[2]. Short-term complications include hyperthermia, new-onset bladder and bowel incontinence, new pressure ulcers, and increased rate of nosocomial infections[5,18]. Severe or permanent injuries include brachial plexus nerve injuries from wrist restraints, joint contractures, and hypoxic encephalopathy[19–22]. Most serious is death from strangulation[23,24].

Obvious physical damage may occur from physical restraints; less appreciated are the psychosocial complications. Strumpf and Evans[25] interviewed elderly patients discharged from the hospital and found significant psychologic distress, with recollections of the restraint experience for up to 6 months after discharge[25].

Others have shown that 20% to 50% of restrained patients demonstrate significant depression, agitation, or anger as a result of restraint[6,26,27].

Additional adverse events are associated with the use of physical restraints, although these are not necessarily a direct cause of the restraint. For example, studies have shown that restrained patients are significantly more likely to die than are nonrestrained patients[4,6,7]. The fact that hospitalized older patients who are restrained are more severely ill and have greater mortality rates calls into question the goals of care and therapy. Clinicians need to weigh the benefits and risks not only of providing therapy, but of administering that therapy in the context of quality care at the end of life[4,28].

NURSES' DECISIONS TO USE PHYSICAL RESTRAINTS

As was true in the long-term-care setting, nurses have been the primary decision makers regarding use of physical restraints in acute care. Although a physician's order is necessary for the use of restraints, hospital nurses typically initiate restraint without consulting physicians[6,29]. Hospital nurses, like nursing home nurses, typically apply physical restraints to prevent patient falls. Surveys of hospital nurses demonstrated that 60% to 77% of restrained patients were put in restraints to prevent falling, 34% to 40% to limit the disruption of therapy, 19% to 23% to keep patients from wandering, 11% to 18% to manage behavioral problems, and 11% to help maintain postural balance[6,25,29]. (It was common for a nurse to cite more than one reason for use of physical restraints. For example, a patient might be restrained to keep from falling and to prevent disruption of therapy.)

Nurses demonstrated considerable variation in the reasons for and decisions about physical restraint. Different nurses often cite varying rationales for the restraint of the same patient; physical restraints are also inconsistently applied from one shift to the next[6,29]. Not only do nurses differ among themselves, but nurses and physicians often disagree with one another about restraint use[29].

ALTERNATIVE APPROACHES TO CARE

Given the numerous reasons and variations in practice, guidelines for any use of physical restraints are unquestionably needed. As part of the Hartford Foundation's Nurses Improving Care of the Hospitalized Elderly (NICHE) Project, a panel of gerontologic nurse experts developed a standard of practice for hospital nurses to follow when considering or applying physical restraint in the care of patients (Box 1). The standard provides background information, assessment parameters, and plan of care, as well as expected outcomes for quality assurance/improvement in meeting JCAHO guidelines. Central to the standard of care is the recommendation that restraints be applied only after exhausting all reasonable alternatives. Thus the standard of practice is nonrestraint, except under exceptional circumstances.

The most important task of the nurse is to identify the underlying reason(s) for the use of restraint. Such a determination forms the basis for identifying alternative approaches to care. For example, if the patient is at risk for falling, factors that place the patient at risk for falling must be identified. In this way, an individualized plan of care is tailored to the patient to minimize the risk of falling. Following is a brief discussion of some alternative approaches in caring for common patient problems that frequently precipitate restraint use. For more detailed information on techniques to reduce the use of physical restraints, excellent references and resources are available for both acute and long-term care[30–32].

Alternatives for Prevention of Falls

Nurses fear that older patients who fall are likely to sustain injury; thus prevention of falls is the most common reason for use of physical restraints in the acute care setting. Falls among hospitalized elders are typically caused by multiple interacting factors that include individual host factors (e.g., unsteady gait), environmental factors (e.g., furniture on wheels), and situational factors (e.g., patient reaching forward)[33]. Fall programs in hospitals and nursing homes typically focus on risks for falling (e.g., the type or

---

BOX 1.   Nursing Standard of Practice Protocol: Use of Mechanical Restraints with Elderly Patients

I.   BACKGROUND
   A. Physical restraint is the use of any manual method or physical or mechanical device that the patient cannot remove, that restricts the patient's physical activity or normal access to his/her body, and that:
      1. Is not a usual and customary part of a medical, diagnostic, or treatment procedure indicated by the patient's medical condition or symptoms.
      2. Does not serve to promote the patient's independent functioning.
   B. The standard of care for hospitalized elderly patients is nonuse of mechanical restraints, except under exceptional circumstances, after all reasonable alternatives have been tried.
   C. Risk factors for use of mechanical restraints in the acute care setting include:
      1. Fall risk.
      2. Tubes or IVs that need stability.
      3. Severe cognitive or physical impairments.
      4. Diagnosis or presence of a psychiatric condition.
      5. Surgery.
   D. Morbidity and mortality risks associated with mechanical restraint use include:
      1. Nerve injury.
      2. New-onset pressure ulcers.
      3. Pneumonia.
      4. Incontinence.
      5. Increased confusion.
      6. Inappropriate drug use.
      7. Strangulation/asphyxiation.
   E. Appropriate alternatives exist to the use of mechanical restraints.
II. ASSESSMENT PARAMETERS
   A. Request information about the use of mechanical restraints from pre-hospital settings.
   B. On admission, identify as "at risk for restraint use" any elderly patient who is agitated, at risk of falling, or disrupting therapy.
   C. Use 1:1 observation or behavior monitor logs to identify and document specific risks. For example, for fall risk, assess impaired cognition, poor balance, impaired gait, orthostatic hypotension, impaired vision and hearing, and the use of sedative and hypnotic agents.
III. CARE STRATEGIES
   A. Prevention:

(continued)

BOX 1. *(continued)*

---

     1. Develop a nursing plan tailored to the patient's presenting problem(s) and specific risk factors.

     2. Consider several alternative interventions. (See bibliography below for suggested alternatives to restraints.)

     3. Refer to occupational and physical therapy for self-care deficits or mobility impairment; use adaptive equipment as appropriate.

     4. Document use and effect of alternatives to restraints.

  B. Treatment:

     1. Use restraints only after exhausting all reasonable alternatives.

     2. When using restraints:

        a. Choose the least restrictive devices.

        b. Reassess the patient's response at least every hour.

        c. Remove restraints every 2 hours.

        d. Renew orders every 24 hours.

     3. Modify the care plan to compensate for the restrictions imposed by restraint use:

        a. Change position frequently and provide skin care.

        b. Provide adequate range of motion.

        c. Assist with ADL, such as eating and use of toilet.

     4. Continue to address underlying condition(s) that prompted restraint use (e.g., gait impairment). Refer to geriatric nurse specialist, occupational or physical therapist, etc., as appropriate.

IV. EVALUATION OF EXPECTED OUTCOMES

  A. Patient: Mechanical restraints will be used only under well-documented exceptional circumstances, after all reasonable alternatives have been tried.

  B. Health care provider: Providers will use a range of interventions other than restraints in the care of patients.

  C. Institution:

     1. Incidence and prevalence of physical restraint use will decrease.

     2. Use of chemical restraints will not increase.

     3. The number of serious injuries related to falls, agitated behavior, and other presenting problems for use of restraints will not increase.

     4. Referrals to occupational and physical therapy will increase, as will availability of adaptive equipment.

     5. Staff will receive ongoing education on the prevention of restraints.

V. FOLLOW-UP TO MONITOR CONDITION

  A. Document incidence of restraint use on an ongoing basis.

(continued)

BOX 1. *(continued)*
B. Educate caregivers to continue assessment and prevention.   C. Identify patient characteristics and care problems that continue to be refractory and involve consultants (geriatric nurse specialist, etc.) in devising an expanded range of alternative approaches.
From References 36–40.

number of risk factors present). Although some interventions may be applied uniformly to all patients (e.g., an available staff member monitoring the unit at all times), other interventions, such as adaptive equipment, are applied to specific patients. The patient at risk must be carefully assessed to identify the specific risk factors for falls and a tailored plan of care initiated.

Patients unable to maintain a sitting posture because of poor trunk muscle strength (e.g., poststroke patients) are sometimes restrained to prevent their sliding out of the chair. Most hospital chairs are straight-backed with an approximately 90-degree sitting angle. Reclining chairs with a modified leg lift maintain the patient's center of gravity in the chair seat. Occupational therapists can help with adaptive cushions (e.g., wedge cushions) or materials that promote sitting in an upright position without restraints.

Patients who demonstrate a weakened or impaired gait are sometimes restrained to prevent unaided walking. Many acute medical and surgical conditions may impair or weaken ambulation. For patients who were independent before hospitalization, an aggressive approach to mobilize them as soon as possible is essential to prevent or minimize functional decline. Consultation with physical therapists early in the course of hospitalization is important. A restorative nursing approach is also essential. For example, instead of relying on bedpans, patients should be encouraged and assisted to walk to the bathroom on a routine basis. Attention also must be paid to room furnishings. Bed height should be at a level to allow the patient's feet to touch the floor while sitting on the edge of the bed. This is difficult when pressure-relieving devices are placed on the mattress. Removal of wheels or replacement with wheels of smaller diameter lowers the bed height.

Patients with a weakened or impaired gait, along with impaired cognition, pose additional challenges to the nursing staff. Those with poor judgment or memory are unlikely to call for assistance before attempting to walk. Close, frequent observation is essential and may be accomplished in several ways: moving the patient closer to the nurses' station; enlisting family or friends to visit, especially during evening or night shifts: use of sitters, companions, or other volunteers; and use of electronic warning devices. Early sounding alarms (e.g., weight-sensitive alarms) are needed for those with both physical and cognitive impairments. (For a more detailed discussion of fall-prevention strategies, refer to Mion and Frengley[32] and Tinetti and Speechley[33].

Alternatives for Protecting or Maintaining Medical Therapy

The second most common reason for use of physical restraints in the hospital setting is to maintain therapy. The nurse must always ask, "Is device necessary?" MacPherson et al.[29] found that nurses and physicians were most likely to restrain patients with medical treatments that they personally had to restart or replace; one must thus conscientiously examine whether a restraint is in place as a matter of convenience. Second, how life-threatening is the removal or disruption of particular medical treatment? Clearly, disruption of a ventilator is much more harmful than disruption of an indwelling bladder catheter. Yet both are often treated the same.

The risks and the benefits of physical restraint must be weighed in maintaining therapy. Are alternative therapies available that might avoid use of physical restraint altogether? For example, if an intravenous line (IV) is needed only for medication, not for fluid replacement, the IV could be replaced by a heparin lock.

Any medical device feels strange to a patient. Simple explanations to the confused patient concerning the device and opportunities for guided exploration are often successful for those with mild confusion. If the treatment device is absolutely necessary, and it appears that the patient will disrupt the therapy, other alternatives may be tried. Strategies for protecting IV lines include use of special gauzes or wraps, arm casings, or long-sleeved hospital gowns or robes to hide or camouflage the insertion site; in addition, IV solution bags or bottles need to be kept behind the patient's field of vision. For more severely demented patients, the latter technique is usually successful. If keeping the IV out of sight is not enough to deter the patient from actively pulling at the insertion site, then mitts (keeping the fingers in a functional extension position rather than tightly flexed) or foam finger extenders (usually obtained through the occupational therapy department) should be tried. In this way, patients still have freedom to use their arms.

Nasogastric tubes used for suction are difficult to maintain in the confused older patient. The tubes cause discomfort and cannot be camouflaged. Explain the tube and necessity of the tube to the patient. If the nagosgastric tube is used for feeding, it may be possible to find alternative routes. It is imperative that speech or occupational therapists evaluate the patient's swallowing as soon as possible. The patient's ability to swallow must be periodically assessed throughout the hospital course. If tube feedings are deemed necessary, then use of percutaneous endoscopic gastrostomy tube should be considered. Because the tube is easily hidden by clothing or abdominal binders, the patient rarely disrupts the device.

Patients who are admitted through the emergency room frequently have indwelling urinary catheters in place. Examination of the need for catheters is essential. Catheters need to be removed as soon as possible because of the morbidity and mortality associated with nosocomial urinary tract infections. If the catheter is truly needed for medical conditions (such as obstruction from benign prostatic hypertrophy), consider whether a straight catheterization routine is medically feasible.

Alternatives to Manage Agitation and Disruptive Behavior

Agitation and disruptive behaviors may occur as a result of delirium, dementia, psychosis, or a combination of these conditions. Depending on the underlying cause, interventions will vary. For example, reality orientation is helpful for treating confusion resulting from delirium and psychosis, but not helpful for confusion resulting from dementia. Consultation from geriatric nurse specialists or psychiatric nurse specialists should be obtained as soon as possible to aid the staff nurse in sorting out the underlying reasons for the confusion and devising a plan of care.

Some general interventions that may be used for all patients with confusion include use of consistent staff; presence of loved ones; limiting the number of personnel and level of noise; judicious use of light, especially at night; and explanations of all procedures. Any underlying conditions causing the agitation or confusion must be treated. Rearranging or combining procedures and treatments so as not to disturb the patient's sleep is important; for example, not waking the patient for vital signs at 1 AM and then waking him or her again for medications at 2 AM. Chemical restraints (i.e., tranquilizers and sedatives) should be used only as a last resort. Keep in mind that use of psychotropic drugs for an already agitated or out-of-control older patient typically does not work quickly. Thus the nurse must exercise caution in repeating doses.

CONCLUSION

Reducing the use of physical restraints in the hospital setting is a complex task and is best accomplished by increasing the staff's awareness and knowledge of alternative methods of care[34,35]. Nurses need not and should not feel alone in taking care of the multiple, intricate problems presented by elderly patients. Professionals in other health care disciplines are available and are valuable in assisting nurses with planning and providing appropriate care to hospitalized elders.

REFERENCES

[1] The Joint Commission 1994 Accreditation Manual for Hospitals; Volume 1. Standards. Oakbrook Terrace, IL: JCAHO; 1993.

[2]   Castle NG, Mor V. Physical restraints in nursing hopes: A review of the literature since the Nursing Home Reform Act of 1987. *Med Care Res Rev.* 1998;55:139–170.

[3]   Bryant H, Fernald L. Nursing Knowledge and use of restraint alternatives: Acute and chronic care. *Geriatr Nurs.* 1997;18(2):57–60.

[4]   Frengley JD, Mion LC. Incidence of physical restraints on acute general medical wards. *J Am Geriatr Soc.* 1986;34:565–568.

[5]   Lofgren RP, MacPherson DS, Granieri R, Myllenbeck S, Sprafka JM. Mechanical restraints on the medical wards: Are protective devices safe? *Am J Public Health.* 1989;79:735–738.

[6]   Mion LC, Frengley JD, Jakovcic CA, Marion JA. A further exploration of the use of physical restraints in hospitalized patients. *J Am Geriatr Soc.* 1989;37:949–956.

[7]   Robbins LJ, Boyko E, Lane J, Cooper D, Jahnigen DW. Binding the elderly: A prospective study of the use of mechanical restraints in an acute care hospital. *J Am Geriatr Soc.* 1987;35:290–296.

[8]   Mion L, Frengley JD, Adams M. Nursing patients 75 years and older. *Nurs Manage.* 1986;17:24–28.

[9]   Warshaw G, Moore J, Friedman S, et al. Functional disability in the hospitalized elderly. *JAMA.* 1982;248:847–850.

[10] Colling J, Park D. Home, safe home. *J Geront Nurs.* 1983;9:175–179.

[11] Gross YT, Shimamoto Y, Rose CL, Frank B. Why do they fall? Monitoring the risk factors in nursing homes. *J Gerontol Nurs.* 1990;16:20–25.

[12] Lund C, Sheafor ML. Is your patient about to fall? *J Gerontol Nurs.* 1985;11:37–41.

[13] Mion LC, Gregor S, Buettner M, Chwirchak D, Lee O, Paras W. Falls in the rehabilitation setting: Incidence and characteristics. *Rehabil Nurs.* 1989;14:17–22.

[14] Walshe A, Rosen H. A study of patient falls from bed. *J Nurs Adm.* 1979;9:31–35.

[15] Wieman HM, Ovear ME. Falls and restraints use in a skilled nursing facility [Abstract]. *J Am Geriatr Soc.* 1986;34:907.

[16] Tinetti ME, Liu WL, Ginter SF. Mechanical restraint use and fall-related injuries among residents of skilled nursing facilities. *Ann Intern Med.* 1992;116:369–374.

[17] Powell C, Mitchell-Pedersen L, Fingerote E, Edmund L. Freedom from restraint: Consequences of reducing physicial restraints in the management of the elderly. *Can Med Assoc J.* 1989;141:561–564.

[18] Miller MB. Iatrogenic and nursigenic effects of prolonged immobilization of the ill aged. *J Am Geriatr Soc.* 1975;23:949–956.

[19] McLardy-Smith P, Burge PD, Watson NA. Ischaemic contracture of

the intrinsic muscles of the hands: A hazard of physical restraint. *J Hand Surg.* 1986;11:65–67.

[20] Berrol S. Risks of restraints in head injury. *Arch Phys Med Rehabil.* 1988;69:537–538.

[21] Scott TE, Gross JA. Brachial plexus injury due to vest restraints [Letter]. *N Engl J Med.* 1989;320:598.

[22] Yob Mo. Use of restraints: Too much or not enough? *Focus Crit Care.* 1988;15:32–33.

[23] Miles SH, Irvine P. Deaths caused by physical restraints. *Gerontologist.* 1992;32:762–766.

[24] Katz L, Weber F, Dodge P. Patient restraint and safety vests: Minimizing the hazards. *Dimens Health Serv.* 1981;58:10–11.

[25] Strumpf NE, Evans LE. Physical restraint of the hospitalized elderly: Perceptions of the patients and nurses. *Nurs Res.* 1988;37:132–137.

[26] Tinetti ME, Liu WL, Marottoli RA, Ginter SF. Mechanical restraint use among residents of skilled nursing facilities: Prevalence, patterns and predictors. *JAMA.* 1991;265:468–471.

[27] Folmar S, Wilson H. Social behavior and physical restraints. *Gerontologist.* 1989;29:650–653.

[28] Evans LK, Strumpf NE. Tying down the elderly: A review of the literature on physical restraint. *J Am Geriatr Soc.* 1989;37:65–74.

[29] MacPherson DS, Lofgren RP, Granieri R, Myllenback S. Deciding to restrain medical patients. *J Am Geriatr Soc.* 1990;38:516–520.

[30] Strumpf N, Wagner J, Evans L, Patterson J. *Reducing Restraints: Individualized Approaches to Behavior.* Huntington Valley, PA: The Whitman Group; 1992.

[31] Braun JV, Lipson S, Eds. *Toward a Restraint-free Environment.* Baltimore: Health Professions Press; 1993.

[32] Mion LC, Frengley JD. Physical restraints in an acute care setting. In: Braun JV, Lipson S, eds. Toward a restraint-free environment. Baltimore: Health Professions Press, 1993.

[33] Tinetti ME, Speechley M. Prevention of falls among the elderly. *N Engl J Med.* 1989;320:1055–1059.

[34] Frengley JD, Mion LC. *Physical Restraint in Acute Hospitals: Routine Physical Restraint: Historical Context and Re-examination of the Practice in Hospitals and Nursing Homes.* Symposium conducted at the 42nd Annual Meeting of the Gerontological Society of America, Minneapolis.

[35] Karlsson S, Bucht G, Sandman PO. Physical restraints in geriatric care. Knowledge, attitudes and use. *Scand J Caring Sci.* 1998;12:48–56.

[36] Evans LK, Strumpf NE, Williams CC. Limiting use of physical restraints: a prerequisite for independent functioning. In Calkins E, Ford A, Katz P, Eds. *The Practice of Geriatrics.* (2nd ed.). Philadelphia: Saunders; 1992.

[37] Mion LC, Frengley JD, Physical restraints in the hospital setting. In Braun JV, Lipson S, Eds. *Toward a restraint free environment.* Baltimore: Baltimore Health Professions Press; 1993.

[38] National Nursing Home Restraint Minimization Program. *Retrain, don't restrain. Field test version: Reference Curriculum.* New York: Jewish Home for the Aged; 1991.

[39] Stilwell EM, Ed. Special issue: Restraints. *J Gerontol Nurs.* 1991;17(2):3–20.

[40] Strumpf N, Wagner J, Evans L, Patterson J. *Reducing restraints: Individualized approaches to behavior.* Huntington Valley, PA: Whitman Group; 1992.

Chapter 13

ADVANCE DIRECTIVES: NURSES HELPING TO PROTECT PATIENT'S RIGHTS

Mathy Mezey, Melissa M. Bottrell, Gloria Ramsey, and the NICHE Faculty

EDUCATIONAL OBJECTIVES:

1. On completion of this chapter, the reader should be able to:
2. Explain what an advance directive is and differentiate between a durable power of attorney and a living will.
3. Describe appropriate assessment parameters to ensure that all patients receive information about advance directives.
4. Describe care strategies to ensure good communication about advance directives with patients and families.Identify outcomes expected from the implementation of this practice protocol.

One of the most difficult situations health care professionals face when caring for elders and other patients is how to assist patients and families trying to make decisions about whether to start, continue, or stop life-sustaining treatments for critically ill patients

Reproduced from Mezey, M, Bottrell, MM, Ramsey G, Advance directives protocol: Nurses helping to protect patients' rights. *Geriatric Nursing,* 1997, 17, 204–210. With permission from Mosby-Year Book, Inc.

and patients who cannot communicate. Elders comprise 73% of deaths each year[1], so end-of-life treatment decisions are more prevalent among this group. Making these decisions can provoke conflict among those involved in caring for patients, including nurses, physicians, social workers, and families. It can be especially difficult when care providers have little knowledge of what care a patient would want or when no one is available to provide such guidance. These decisions can also be more difficult with elderly persons because about 30% of the elderly do not have a relative or friend who can make care decisions for them. Health care professionals, especially nurses, can improve end-of-life decision making for elderly patients by encouraging the use of advance directives, which can provide guidance with regard to the patient's treatment decisions for a patient who lacks decision-making capacity[2]. Nurses may also be legally responsible for discussing advance directives with patients depending on the care setting in which they work.

This chapter summarizes the literature as it relates to the nurses' roles in informing patients about advance directives and in supporting patient's treatment decisions. The care protocol included at the end of this chapter serves as a guide for nurses in all practice settings who want guidelines for how to help patients get their end-of-life care wishes followed.

With congressional passage of the Patient Self Determination Act in 1991[3], more health care professionals have come into contact with advance directives. This act requires all facilities that receive Medicare or Medicaid funds to inform patients, on admission, of their rights under state law to make health care decisions, including their options to complete an advance directive. However, the basis for advance directives has a much longer history. Predicated on the Western tradition of the importance of individual freedom and choice, also called the principal of autonomy, individuals have a moral right to make decisions about their own treatment. Furthermore, the New Jersey Supreme Court determined that competent individuals also have the constitutional right to accept or reject medical treatment under the right of privacy[4]. This right was supported by the U.S. Supreme court in the matter of Nancy Cruzan[5], a nationally recognized case that brought the issue of an individual's right to terminate unwanted treatment into the public eye.

Most states, with the exception of New York, Massachusetts and Michigan, have statutes regarding the legal basis for living wills, a type of advance directive. The statutes usually outline the conditions under which an advance directive is legally valid and when it should be followed. In spite of the various justifications and legal protections for the individual's right to make decisions about their own care, it is difficult to protect a patient's right to autonomy when the person is unable to communicate due to mental or physical incapacity. It is these situations that advance directives can improve by:

1. Allowing individuals to provide directions about the kind of medical care they do or do not want if they become unable to make decisions or communicate their wishes.
2. Providing guidance for health care professionals and families with regard to how to make health care decisions that reflect the person's wishes should that person be unable to make health care decisions.
3. Providing immunity for health care professionals and families from civil and criminal liability when health care professionals follow the advance directive in good faith and respect the applicable state statute regarding advance directives.

TYPES OF ADVANCE DIRECTIVES

Two types of advance-directive documents are available: durable power of attorney for health care (also called a health care proxy) and living wills. A durable power of attorney for health care allows an individual to appoint someone, called a health care proxy, agent or surrogate, to make health care decisions if the individual loses the ability to make decisions or communicate his/her wishes. The health care proxy has the authority to interpret the patient's wishes on the basis of the medical circumstances of the situation and is not restricted to deciding only if life-sustaining treatment can be withdrawn or withheld. Thus the proxy can make decisions as the need arises, and such decisions can respond directly to the decision at hand rather than being restricted only to circumstances that were thought of previously. Designating a health care proxy is preferable to completing a living will because it appoints one person to speak for the patient. Although most states have family consent laws that designate which family member can make decisions for incompetent patients, it is often unclear how to resolve disputes between family members who bear the same relationship to the patient. Designating a proxy can overcome this problem and is especially important when an individual chooses not to appoint a family member. For elderly patients who do not have a family member or friend that could be a proxy, however, completing a living will that outlines their wishes is preferable to not providing any information about care preferences.

A living will provides specific instructions to health care providers about particular kinds of health care treatment an individual would or would not want to prolong life. Living wills are often used to declare a wish to refuse, limit, or withhold life-sustaining treatment when an individual is unable to communicate. They may also be used to give instructions about what kind of treatment an individual would want administered, although no cases have been reported where a living will has been used to request treatment considered futile by health care providers. All but three states (New York, Massachusetts, and Michigan) have detailed statutes recognizing living wills. The usefulness of living wills is limited, however to those circumstances that were thought of before the person became incapable of making decisions. If a situation occurs that the living will does not address, providers and families may not know how to proceed and still respect the patient's wishes. Appointing a health care proxy can assist in these circumstances.

Some state statutes also allow a combined directive that includes elements of both a living will and an health care proxy in one document. A combined document is superior to a living will or health care proxy because if the patient's instructions do not apply to the situation at hand, either because they are too general or too specific, the designated proxy can provide the additional background and authority that families and health care providers need to make the right decision for the patient. Furthermore, the instructions in the living will portion can guide the proxy when making decisions for an incompetent patient.

Although they prefer written advance directives, the courts do respect oral advance directives, especially in emergency situations, and have relied on them in deciding to forego life-sustaining treatment. The issues courts have considered when determining whether an oral advance directive was valid include whether the statement was made on a serious or solemn occasion, consistently repeated, made by a mature person who understood the underlying issues, consistent with the values demonstrated in the other aspects of the patient's life (including the patient's religion), made just before the need for the treatment decision, and specifically addressed the actual condition of the patient. Such issues should be discussed and documented by health care providers when discussing advance directives with patients.

NURSES' ROLES IN ADVANCE DIRECTIVES

Nurses play an important role in introducing patients to information about advance directives and helping patients complete them[2]. Although surveys of the general public report positive attitudes toward advance directives, few patients actually have completed one. Even patients at higher risk of becoming incapable of making decisions and who, therefore, might be more likely to need one are not necessarily more likely to complete one. Completion of an advance directive is more concentrated among White patients with higher education and income levels.

Evidence suggests that talking with patients about advance directives can change this picture. For instance, patients participating in educational interventions in which they had regular conversations with their health care provider about advance directives were more likely to complete a directive[6]. Nurses should not wait for the patient to broach the subject. Patients want to discuss end-of-life care and living wills[7], but they expect providers to initiate these discussions. For patients who find it difficult to initiate such discussions with their families, the nurse can provide a format for discussions, help ensure that the conversation is comprehensive, and use advance directives to minimize disagreements between patients and their families. Patients often state that they complete advance directives to ease their family's financial and emotional burden and to ease decision making. Nurses can encourage this use of the document.

All patients should be approached regarding whether they have already completed an advance directive document, whether they have already received information about advanced directives or whether they would like assistance in completing one. This should occur during the early stages of an admission and during a regularly scheduled appointment. If the patient has completed an advance directive, the care provider responsible for the patient's care should review the directive with the patient to understand its contents and ascertain whether the information is current. A copy of that directive should be placed in the patient's chart where it is easily accessible by all care providers. If the patient has designated a health care proxy, the provider should ascertain whether the proxy has a copy of the document as well.

Patients who have not completed an advance directive should be asked if they would like to discuss advance directives and offered written information about advance directives. Care providers should assist patients who subsequently wish to complete a directive. The completed advance directive should be placed in the patient's chart where it is easily accessible by responsible care providers and be reviewed with the patient's regular physician, if one is available, and a copy should be provided to the health care proxy if one is designated.

It is important that all adult patients, regardless of their demographic characteristics such as sex, religion, socioeconomic status, diagnosis, or prognosis be approached to discuss advance directives. Discussions should also be translated into the patient's preferred language to enable all patients to get information about advance directives. Evidence suggests that patients from certain demographic groups are less likely to be approached about advance directives or be provided with information about them[8]. Lack of information may be one reason why people with less education or lower income or who are Black or Hispanic are less likely to formulate advance directives[8–10]. Transmitting information in a manner that is readily understood is the first element of informed decision making. Failure to transmit information in a meaningful way, for example, failing to take into account the hearing and visual deficits of some older people, can result in the erroneous conclusion on the part of health care professionals that the person lacks the capacity to execute an advance directive. All patients have a legal right to get information about advance directives so that their treatment wishes can be followed.

CULTURAL ISSUES AND ADVANCE DIRECTIVES

It is important to be sensitive to various cultural issues that can arise when discussing end-of-life care, including different concepts of autonomy or decision-making structures within a family. For some individuals, an advance directive may conflict directly with behavioral norms or the decision-making process identified by their culture. For others, especially those persons whose access to regular medical care is limited by economic issues or social status, limiting medical care in any way would seem unnecessary because they have too little, not too much, health care. Those who have experienced discrimination throughout their lives also may distrust the intent of health care providers with respect to advance directives. Also certain cultural factors in non-White communities may prohibit discussions of death and dying, for example, fears among Black people that Acquired Immune Deficiency Syndrome was developed to wipe out the community[11]. These cultural issues do not mean that individuals do not want information about advance directives or end-of-life decision making; instead the subject should be approached in a culturally sensitive manner by health care providers.

DECISION-MAKING CAPACITY TO EXECUTE A DIRECTIVE

Of special consideration when trying to decide who should be approached about advance directives is the patient's capacity to make decisions about his or her health care. A patient's inability to make financial decisions or communicate verbally does not mean that they cannot communicate important information about their care preferences.

The issue of informing residents in nursing homes about advanced directives warrants some special consideration. In nursing homes, residents perceived to have the requisite cognitive ability almost always have the opportunity to discuss advance directives, usually with a social worker and sometimes with a nurse or physician. On the other hand, nursing home residents who are perceived by staff to lack the capacity to understand advance directives are not given the opportunity to discuss advance directives. Unfortunately, the determination that a resident can't engage in a discussion about advance directives is not always based on an assessment of a resident's capacity. Thus there is a risk that residents with communication disorders or those with minimal dementia may not be provided with an opportunity to appoint a health care proxy or to execute a living will. It is recommended that all residents, with the exception of residents who are comatose or have very advanced dementia, be given the opportunity to talk with a health care provider about executing a health care proxy.

CREATING A FAVORABLE CLIMATE FOR ADVANCE DIRECTIVE DISCUSSION

There are several ways to create an environment that is conducive to positive discussions about end-of-life decision making and advance directives, such as choosing the appropriate timing and location of such discussions. Timing of the discussion is important; an acute episode or emergency admission is an inappropriate time to receive information about advance directives. Patients may be more receptive to information about advance directives if they receive it in a preadmission package to read at home or as part of the discharge process when the impact of hospitalization is still fresh, but without the distraction of acute symptoms and paperwork. Having information provided by an attending physician or nurse at a regular office visit or by a regular care provider when the patient is in the nursing home may also improve these discussions.

Some patients may be reluctant to discuss end-of-life care planning and advance directives because they are reluctant to discuss their own death. Hare and Nelson[12] reported that 38% of patients (n = 167, 45 patients age 65 years or older) were "interested and eager" to discuss a living will, 32% were "interested and willing, but not eager," 23% were "uninterested and somewhat resistant," and 7% were "openly resistant" to discussions of advance directives. Elpern et al.[13] found that 44% of patients (n = 96, range 25 to 88 years, median age 57.5) thought it "depressing to think about dying." Education and information about advance directives may not completely counteract the discomfort associated with discussing death and dying. But nurses and other health care professionals need to learn techniques to discuss death realistically and sensitively with patients and their families. These techniques include becoming aware of the spiritual needs of patients and including other professionals, such as the clergy, in discussions about end-of-life issues[14].

Each person's right not to complete an advance directive should also be respected. Inform patients that neither providers nor the facility will abandon them or provide substandard care if the patient elects to formulate an advance directive. However, if the patient chooses not to discuss the issue for whatever reason, note that desire in the patient's chart and accept the patient's wishes.

NURSES' PERSPECTIVES ON ADVANCE DIRECTIVES

Health care providers raise a number of issues when they express negative feelings about advance directives. Some may mistrust the validity of the information contained in the advance directive because they believe or fear that the patient did not fully understand the advance directives' content or purpose[15]. The ability to predict specific treatment choices based upon generally stated beliefs is not uniformly congruent for patients and their proxies[16–18]. Overall, however, even if flawed, patients' wishes (as spelled out in living wills) and decisions of health care proxies are more likely to approximate the patient's own treatment preferences than the decisions of others. In general, patients' decisions seem to be fairly stable over time, especially among patients who have completed advance directives[19,20].

Providers are often hesitant to approach patients about directives when the issue of stopping or withdrawing treatment is imminent[21]. Many providers erroneously believe that there is a legal difference between forgoing and discontinuing treatments, including nutrition and hydration[22]. A patient has a legal and ethical right to discontinue nutrition and hydration; however, the legal evidence and procedures required to forgo or discontinue this treatment vary by state. Nurses should be aware of their state law regarding forgoing or withdrawing nutrition and hydration. Nurses should also be aware of their own moral biases toward providing nutrition and hydration and should remember that there is no legal basis for discriminating against a patient on the basis of their choice to ask for or reject treatments, including nutrition and hydration.

It is important to know the facility's method for resolving conflicts between family members and the patient, the patient/family and care providers, or between health care professionals. If a patient or proxy's treatment choice conflicts with a nurse's beliefs and the nurse cannot offer care in accordance with those wishes, the appropriate person within the facility should be notified. The overriding concern should be that the patient's care wishes be followed. Patients should be cared for by a nurse who can follow their wishes or the patient should be transferred to another facility.

EDUCATION

Education is an important component in changing providers' comfort with and willingness to approach patients about advance directives. When nurses are well informed, they are more comfortable with such discussions and have more discussions with their patients, and their patients complete more advance directives than do patients of uneducated providers[10,23,24]. However, thorough education requires more than a description of the law and steps in formulating directives. Nurses need to learn how to discuss advanced care planning with patients and families, assess decisional capacity to execute an advance directive, identify methods to help patients analyze benefits and burdens of decisions, and resolve conflicts among staff with different values and beliefs about end-of-life treatment. Nurses should learn guidelines for treatments often encountered during end-of-life care, information about the psychology of decision making and develop a dialogue between those in a facility that make ethical recommendations and those who carry them out at the bedside[21].

EVALUATION OF IMPLEMENTING THE ADVANCE DIRECTIVES PROTOCOL

To determine whether care practice regarding discussions of advance directives has changed after implementation of this protocol, personnel can measure whether the following changes occurred in the facility: the percentage of patients who have been asked about advance directives increased; all charts note whether a patient does or does not have an advance directive; the percentage of advance directives included in patient charts increased; the percentage of nurses and other staff who are comfortable or satisfied with the role of advance directives in patient care decisions increased; or whether more staff were asked to assist patients in executing advance directives.

GERIATRIC NURSING STANDARD OF PRACTICE:
ADVANCE DIRECTIVES PROTOCOL

Guiding Principals:
1. All people have the right to decide what will be done with their bodies.
2. All individuals are presumed to have decision-making capacity until deemed otherwise.
3. All patients who can participate in a conversation, either verbally or through alternate means of communication, should be approached to discuss advance directives.

GERIATRIC NURSING STANDARD OF PRACTICE: *(continued)*

I. BACKGROUND
    A. Decisions about stopping treatment are more prevalent among the elderly. The elderly compose 73% of deaths each year[1]. Health care professionals can improve the end-of-life decision making for elderly patients by encouraging the use of advance directives.

    Advance directives have three functions:
    1. To allow individuals to provide directions about the kind of medical care they do or do not want if they become unable to make decisions or communicate their wishes.
    2. To provide guidance for health care professionals and families as to how to make health care decisions that reflect the person's wishes should that person be unable to make decisions.
    3. To provide immunity for health care professionals and families from civil and criminal liability when health care professionals follow the advance directive in good faith and respect the applicable state statute regarding advance directives.
    B. Advance directives are of two types: Durable Power of Attorney for Health Care (also called a health care proxy) and living will.
        1. A *Durable Power of Attorney* allows an individual to appoint someone, called a health care proxy, agent, or surrogate, to make health care decisions for him or her should he or she lose the ability to make decisions or communicate his or her wishes.
        2. A *living will* provides specific instructions to health care providers about particular kinds of health care treatment an individual would or would not want to prolong life. Living wills are often used to declare a wish to refuse, limit, or withhold life-sustaining treatment when an individual is unable to communicate.
    C. Nurses can make a difference in whether a patient completes an advance directive:
        1. Patients uniformly state that they want more information about advance directives
        2. Patients want nurses (and doctors) to approach them about advance directives.
        3. Fewer than 20% of Americans have completed an advance directive.
        4. Patients who are non-White, have less education, or are from lower income levels are less likely to have executed an advance directive. These patients are also the most likely to state that they were not approached to discuss end-of-life decisions.

(continued)

GERIATRIC NURSING STANDARD OF PRACTICE: *(continued)*

II. ASSESSMENT PARAMETERS
   A. All patients (with the exception of patients with PVS, severe dementia, or coma) should be approached soon after their admission to determine if they have a living will or if they have designated a proxy.
   B. All patients, regardless of their demographic characteristics such as age, gender, religion, socioeconomic status, diagnosis, or prognosis should be approached to discuss advance directives.
   C. Discussions about advance directives should be translated into the patient's preferred language to enable all patients to get information about advance directives.
   D. Patients who have been determined to lack capacity to make other decisions may still have the capacity to designate a proxy or make health care decisions. Decision-making capacity should be determined for each individual based on whether the patient has the ability to make the specific decision in question.
   E. If a living will or proxy has <u>not</u> been executed:
      1. Give the patient written information about advance directives.
      2. Have a conversation with the patient about advance directives.
      3. Help the patient to execute an advance directive if requested.
      4. Place a completed document in the patient's chart and make it available to the attending physician/nurse and the health care proxy.
   F. If a living will has been completed or proxy <u>has</u> been designated:
      1. Is that document easily available on the patient's chart and located near the patient, i.e. not in the records department?
      2. Does the attending physician/nurse know of its existence and have a copy? Did the attending physician/nurse review the document to ascertain if the stated wishes still reflect the patient's wishes?
      3. Does the designated health care proxy have a copy of the document?
      4. Has the document been recently reviewed by the patient, attending physician/nurse and the proxy?
   G. Oral Advance Directives (verbal directives) are allowed in some states if there is clear and convincing evidence of the patient's wishes. Clear and convincing evidence can include evidence that the patient has a significant relationship with the health care provider or the wish was repeated over time. Legal rules surrounding oral advance directives vary by state.
III. CARE STRATEGIES
   A. Open the discussion about advance directives with patients and families. Nurses can assist patients and families trying to deal with end-of-life care issues.

(continued)

GERIATRIC NURSING STANDARD OF PRACTICE: *(continued)*

  B. Patients who may be reluctant to discuss their own mortality or accept their current health situation, may be willing to discuss these issues with a nurse if not a doctor.

  C. Assess each patient's need for and ability to cope with the information provided. Patients from other cultures may not subscribe to Western notions of autonomy, but that does not mean that these patients do not want this information or that they would not have conversations with their families if the issue was discussed by their nurse.

  D. Be sensitive to race, culture, ethnicity, and religion when discussing end-of-life care issues. A patient's feelings about these issues can substantially influence decisions to complete an advance directive.

  E. Race, culture, ethnicity, and religion may impact the health care decision-making process and nurses should be mindful of these but always treat the patient as an individual, not as a class of persons.

  F. Be sensitive to each patient's fears about his or her own mortality and involve other professionals, including clergy, if desired by the patient in discussions about advance directives.

  G. Respect each person's right not to complete an advance directive.

  H. Inform patients that you will not abandon them or provide substandard care if they elect to formulate an advance directive.

  I. Know the hospital's method of resolving conflicts between family members and the patient or patient/family and care providers. This may include consultation from social work or the patient advocate or bringing the issue to the hospital ethics committee.

  J. Notify the appropriate persons if you are unable to provide care should the patient's wishes conflict with your beliefs.

IV. Evaluation of Expected Outcomes

To determine if practice regarding discussions of advance directive has changed note whether:

  A. The percentage of patients asked about advance directives in the hospital increased.

  B. All charts note whether the patient does or does not have an advance directive.

  C. When a patient has an advance directive, the advance directives is included in the patient's chart.

  D. The number of nurses and other staff who are comfortable satisfied with the role of advance directives in patient care decisions increased.

  E. More staff were asked to assist patients in executing advance directives.

REFERENCES

[1] U.S. Department of Health and Human Services. Annual Summary of Births, Marriages, Divorces and Deaths: United States, 1994. *Monthly Vital Statistics Report.* 1995:43(13).

[2] Kirmse JM. Aggressive implementation of advance directives. *Crit Can Nurs Q.* 1998;21(1):83–89.

[3] Pub. L. No. 101–508, §4206, 4751 [hereinafter OBRA], 104 stat. 1388–115 to 117, 1388–204 to 206 (codified at 42 U.S.C.A. §1395cc(f) (1) & id. §1396a(a) (West Supp. 1994)

[4] 70 N.J. 10, 335 A.2d 647, cert. den., 429 U.S. 922 (1976)

[5] Cruzan v. Director, 497 U.S. 261, 100 (S. Ct. 1990) 2841, 111 L. Ed. 2d 224.

[6] Luptak MK, Bould C. A method for increasing elders' use of advance directives. *Gerontologist.* 1994;34:409–412.

[7] Emanuel LL, Barry MJ, Stoeckle JD, Ettelson LM, Emanuel EJ. Advanced directives for medical care: A case for greater use. *N Engl J Med.* 1991;324:889–895.

[8] Mezey M, Ramsey G, Mitty E, Leitman R, Rapporport M. Patient Self Determination Act (PSDA): cultural and socioeconomic differences among recently discharged hospital patients. Presented at the American Public Health Association 123rd Annual Meeting, November 1, 1995, San Diego, CA.

[9] High DM. Advance directives and the elderly: A study of intervention strategies to increase use. *Gerontologist.* 1993;33:342–349.

[10] Robinson MK, DeHaven MJ, Kock KA. Effects of the patient self-determination act on patient knowledge and behavior. *J Fam Prac.* 1993;37:363–368.

[11] Hass JS, Weissman JS, Cleary PD, et. al. Discussions of preferences for life sustaining care by persons with AIDS. *Arch Int Prn Med.* 1993;153:1241–1248.

[12] Hare J, Nelson C. Will outpatients complete living wills? *J Gen Int Med.* 1991;6:41–46.

[13] Elpern EH, Yellen SB, Burton LA. A preliminary investigation of opinions and behaviors regarding advance directives for medical care. *Am J Crit Care.* 1993;2:161–167.

[14] Basile CM. Advance directives and advocacy in end of life decisions. *Nurse Pract.* 1998;23(5):44–46.

[15] Jacobsen JA, White BE, Battin MP, Francis LP, Green DJ, Kansworm ES. Patients' understanding and use of advance directives. *West J Med.* 1994;160:232–236.

[16] Emanuel EJ, Weinberg DS, Gonin RG, Hummel LR, Emanuel LL.

How well is the patient self-determination act working? An early assessment 95. *Am J Med.* 1993;619.

[17] Uhlmann RF, Pearlman RA, Cain KC. Physicians' and spouses; predictions of elderly patients' resuscitation preferences. *J Gerontol.* 1988;43:115–121.

[18] Schneiderman LJ, Pearlman RA, Kaplan RM, Anderson JP, Rosenberg EM. Relationship of general advance directive instructions to specific life-sustaining treatment preferences in patients with serious illness. *Arch Intern Med.* 1992;152:2114–2122.

[19] Emanuel LL, Emanuel EJ, Toeckle JD, Hummel LR, Barry MJ. Advance directives: Stability of patient's treatment choices. *Arch Intern Med.* 1994;154:209–217.

[20] Danis M, Garret J, Harris R, Patrick DL. Stability of choices about life-sustaining treatments. *Ann Intern Med.* 1994;120:567–573.

[21] Solomon MZ, O'Donnell L, Jennings B, et al. Decisions near the end of life: professional views on life-sustaining treatments. *Am J Publ Health.* 1993;83:14–23.

[22] Olson E. Ethical issues in the nursing home. *Mt Sinai J Med.* 1993;60:555–559.

[23] Greenberg JM, Doblin BH, Shapiro DW, Linn LS, Wenger NS. Effect of an educational program on medical student's conversations with patients about advance directives. *J Gen Int Med.* 1993;8:683–685.

[24] Richter J, Eisemann M, Bauer B, Kribeck H. Decisions and attitudes of nurses in the care of chronically ill elderly patients. *Pflege.* 1998;11(2):96–99.

Chapter 14

DISCHARGE PLANNING AND HOME FOLLOW-UP OF ELDERS

Roberta L. Campbell, Mary D. Naylor, and the NICHE Faculty

EDUCATIONAL OBJECTIVES:

At the completion of this chapter, the reader should be able to:
1. State at least one assessment parameter for discharge planning in each of the following areas: physical health, medication regimen, functional status, follow-up health care, and safety.
2. Identify situations in which it is important to include caregivers or family members in teaching sessions.
3. Translate assessment findings into specific care strategies for maximum recovery of function.

In 1997, of the 38.6 million aged & disabled Americans who were enrolled in Medicare, 3.9 million (10%) received home care services[1]. Almost all of these services follow a hospitalization and are aimed at rehabilitating patients to their highest level of function and health. The 18,000+ home care agencies make close to 280 million visits to 3.9 million Medicare enrollees at a cost of over $18 billion. Making best use of home care rehabilitative services requires close coordination and discharge planning between the hospital and the home care agency.

Planning for the return home of a hospitalized older adult must consider the patient's and family's capabilities prior to admission, the patient preferences, and the resources needed for recovery[2–9]. Appropriate planning begins on the patient's admission to the hospital and continues into the home. Information is obtained from the patient and/or family about the reason for hospitalization, the medication regimen, prior functional ability, and the perceived need for home services. Areas for nursing assessment include health problems, medication regimen, functional status, necessary assistive devices, and safety. Early identification of needs will prevent unnecessary delays in discharge, facilitate referral for rehabilitative services, and provide time for patient education[8,10]. Although whole effective home-care strategies are based on interdisciplinary planning, patient/family goals must guide decisions. Evaluation of the outcomes of care include quality, access, cost-effectiveness, and patient/family satisfaction.

ASSESSMENT

One of the first items to consider is the patient's self-rating of overall health[2,7,11]. This subjective indication of the patient's response to illness is an indicator of the perceived need for follow-up intervention. The nurse would also assess the impact of the health problem(s) that resulted in the hospitalization (see Box 1). If the patient has a referring or admitting health care provider, the history of how the problem has been managed should be obtained. The patient's response to the health problem, including the nature and duration of symptoms, interference with daily functioning, effectiveness of actions taken to relieve the symptoms, and availability of friends and family to provide support are important factors in planning for the return home. It is necessary to ascertain early on who will be the designated coordinator of post-discharge care.

The medication regimen is the second assessment area. Assess

BOX 1. Planning Home Care Rehabilitation Needs	
Processes of care	Strategies
Health problems	Self-perception of health
	Presenting symptoms
	Physical, psychological, emotional, social, and economic response to health problem(s)
	Adherence to medical regimen
	Effectiveness of treatment
	Knowledge of disease process and management of symptoms
Medication regimen	Knowledge of medications schedule and purpose
	Use of over-the-counter medications
	Need for assistance/compliance aid
	Problem obtaining medications
	Visual/dexterity limitations
	Complexity of regimen
Functional status	Limitations in activities of daily living
	Actual or potential deficits related to acute illness or treatment regimen
	Limitations in instrumental activities
	Availability and adequacy of support system
	Imposed activity restrictions during recovery period
	Transportation to obtain necessary services
	Availability of assistive devices
Follow-up health care	Name and telephone number of care providers
	Appropriate access to services
	Name and telephone number of home care agency
	Patient satisfaction with health care services
Safety	Adequate home ventilation and lighting
	Physical layout of home: entry, stairs, bathroom access, meal preparation
	Telephone access
	Knowledge of emergency exits
	Safe use of medical equipment
	Neighborhood safety

the patient's medication knowledge, degree of independence in medication administration, and adherence to prescribed regimen[3,7,12]. Discuss the use of over-the-counter medications[13]. Find out if the patient needs assistance with medication administration or if a compliance aid is used as a reminder. Problems obtaining the medication, such as inadequate financial resources or transportation barriers, must be addressed. If the patient brought medications from home, examine labels for possible misunderstandings. For example, does the patient refer to the medication by the generic name, or simply by its expected action? Does the prescribed dosage match the strength of the pill in the container, or does the patient have to make some adjustment, that is, cut the pill in half or double the dose on appropriate days? The baseline understanding of the medications by the caregiver(s) should be assessed as well. Caregivers should always be included in teaching sessions[3]. Modification of the dosing schedule may be needed to ensure the highest level of patient independence.

An assessment of functional status in terms of activities of daily living (ADLs such as eating, bathing and grooming, toileting, dressing, transfers, and walking) should include the expected impact of the health problem(s) on performance of daily activities[6,13–16]. Deficits resulting from the acute health problem or the treatment regimen must also be considered. Assessments by physical and occupational therapists will help determine recovery potential. Patients and families need to be instructed in the use of any assistive devices or medical equipment.

Instrumental activities of daily living (IADLs) should also be assessed[16–18]. Individuals may need assistance with meal preparation, homemaking, shopping, and transportation. It is important to identify specific caregivers and the specific tasks they are willing to perform. If it is anticipated that the patient's care needs will be greater than the level of available support, the patient and family will need assistance in making alternative arrangements. Limitations in some activities, such as stair climbing, may necessitate the need for a portable toilet or a hospital bed on the first floor of the home.

It is important to assess availability of transportation for follow-up medical care. Transportation problems can result in missed appointments, lack of follow-up monitoring, inappropriate use of emergency services, and poor recovery.

Services provided prior to hospitalization must be reviewed and providers notified[18]. A medical social worker will need to be involved if multiple services were in place. If the services are satisfactory and remain necessary, the agency should be informed prior to patient discharge in order to schedule the resumption of services.

Safety in the home should always be assessed[6,13]. Questions about the physical layout of the home, the presence of stairs, adequate ventilation and lighting, bathroom facilities, facilities for preparation and storage of meals, access to a telephone, and emergency exits are often overlooked. The need for medical equipment, including a cane, walker, shower seat, portable toilet, raised toilet seat, grab bars, or handrail on stairs and other assistive devices must be addressed. If the patient will be alone in the home for periods of time provisions must be made for toileting safely, changing body positions, obtaining food and water, and accessing emergency care.

CARE STRATEGIES

Successful rehabilitation requires specific objectives for ensuring continuity of care, appropriate use of health provider's expertise, and coordination of services toward promotion of a maximum level of functioning[14,19]. A multidisciplinary team approach with patient and family input has the best chance of success[4,6,13–14,16,20]. Early planning, including an interdisciplinary discharge planning record, can increase patient and family satisfaction with care, prevent delays at time of discharge, and allow time to explore care options (see Box 2).

Communication among disciplines is facilitated by formal processes such as interdisciplinary care planning and documentation, unit-based assignments for discharge planners, and liaisons to community agencies[4–5,9,17–18]. An interdisciplinary record can serve multiple purposes including communication of the patient's discharge needs, identification of and referral to appropriate providers, and documentation of patient and caregiver education.

With decreased lengths of hospital stays, it is important that referrals for home and community services be initiated early[8]. In many hospitals, discharge planning has been incorporated into critical pathways that are used to guide clinical decision making for patients admitted with specific diseases[19]. Nurses must be

BOX 2. Care Strategies for Discharge Planning	
Processes of care	Strategies
Communications of assessment findings	Begin communicating discharge needs at the time of admission
	Make referrals as needed
	Document on interdisciplinary records
	Participate in unit-based discharge planning rounds
	Discuss simplification of medication regimen
	Eliminate communication barriers
Designing the plan	Involve patient and family
	Get a multidisciplinary perspective on treatment options
Patient/family teaching	Formulate learning objectives based on assessment findings
	Plan teaching sessions with patient & care giver
	Provide verbal and written instruction
	Begin teaching as soon as patient is ready to learn
	Plan sessions within the anticipated length of stay
	Give clear, concise directions about symptom management
	Prepare and discuss a medication chart
	Suggest self-care measures to prevent problems and maintain health
	Prepare and review the discharge instruction sheet with the patient and family
Monitoring/evaluation	Monitor hospital course and treatment response
	Follow critical pathway guidelines for length of stay and resource use
	Document reason for variance from pathway
	Prevent iatrogenic complications
	Delegate appropriately
	Reduce barriers to delivery of care
	Evaluate patient/family satisfaction with care
	Monitor postdischarge follow-up care

familiar with these pathways in order to assure that patients are prepared for discharge within the projected time frame or that justifications for a longer stay associated with the discharge needs of patients are explicitly identified[21].

An individualized patient instruction sheet should be prepared and reviewed with the patient and family prior to discharge. This form should provide the patient and care providers with instructions to promote continuity of care[22]. Special instructions assist the patient and family with monitoring and reporting health problems, and with medications and treatment schedules. Patients should be given the names and phone numbers of the home care agency and involved service providers as well as emergency numbers that may be needed.

Having a consistent nurse caregiver, especially an advanced practice gerontological nurse who cares for the elderly patients in the hospital and then follows them at home for a period of several weeks, has been shown to decrease complications after discharge and prevent unnecessary readmission to the hospital[2]. These nurses used their advanced knowledge and skills to provide direct care to patients and caregivers and coordinate the services provided by others[23]. Because these nurses have gotten to know patients and their needs while hospitalized, they are able to prevent or identify complications quickly when the patient is at home, reinforce patient and family teaching begun in the hospital, and recommend to the physician essential modifications in the treatment plan.

EVALUATIONS OF OUTCOME

An evaluation of outcomes should include the three areas of access, quality, and cost-effectiveness of care[2,5,24–25]. Assessment of the extent to which patients are informed about available resources to meet their needs, offered choice in providers and settings for service delivery, and understand the financial implications of these choices should be completed[9,26]. Patients' and caregivers' satisfaction with services and suggestions for improvement should be elicited. Assessment of the progress made by patients and outcomes should be conducted[2,6,11]. The extent to which the services provided promoted positive outcomes and prevented or minimized the use of more costly postdischarge services should be determined[2,5,23]. Quality discharge planning and home follow-up thus becomes delivering the right service at the right time for the right price.

ACKNOWLEDGMENT

Supported by a Grant from the National Institute of Nursing Research (NR02095–07).

REFERENCES

[1] Research Department. *Basic statistics about home care;* National Association for Home Care, November 1997; Washington, DC: National Association for Home Care.

[2] Naylor MD, Brooten D, Jones R, Lavizzo-Mourey R, Mezey M, Pauly M. Comprehensive discharge planning for the hospitalized elderly: A randomized clinical trial. *Ann Intern Med.* 1994;120:999–1006.

[3] Reiley P, Iezzoni LI, Phillips R, Davis RB, Tuchin LI, Calkins D. Discharge planning: Comparison of patients' and nurses' perceptions of patients following hospital discharge. *Image: J Nsg Scholarship.* 1996;28:143–147.

[4] Pilcher MW. Post-discharge care: How to follow up. *Nursing 86.* 1986;16:50–51.

[5] Proctor EK, Morrow-Howell N, Kaplan SJ. Implementation of discharge plans for chronically ill elders discharged home. *Hlth Soc Work.* 1996;21(1):30–40.

[6] Zarle NC. Continuity of care: Balancing care of elders between health care settings. *Nsg Clinics NA.* 1989;24(3):697–705.

[7] Kennedy L, Neidlinger S, Scroggins K. Effective comprehensive discharge planning for hospitalized elderly. *Gerontologist.* 1989;27:577–580.

[8] Johnson J. Where's discharge planning on your list? *Geriatr Nurs.* 1989;9(3):148–149.

[9]   Bull MJ. Patients' and professionals' perceptions of quality in discharge planning. *J Nurs Care Qual.* 1994;8(2):47–61.

[10] Wacker RR, Kundrat MA, Keith PM. What do discharge planners plan? Implications for older Medicare patients. *J Applied Geront.* 1991;10:197–207.

[11] Johnson N, Fethke CC. Postdischarge outcomes and care planning for the hospitalized elderly. In: McClelland E, Kelly K, Buckwalter KC, Eds. *Continuity of care: Advancing the concept of discharge planning.* New York: Grune & Stratton; 1985:229–239.

[12] Schneider JK, Hornberger S, Booker J, Davis A, Kralicek R. A medication discharge planning program. *Clin Nsg Res.* 1993;2(1):41–53.

[13] Dugan J, Mosel L. Patients in acute care settings. Which health care services are provided? *J Geront Nsg.* 1992;18(7):31–36.

[14] Kresevic DM, Mezey M, NICHE faculty. Assessment of function: Critically important to acute care of elders. *Geriatr Nurs.* 1997;18(5): 216–222.

[15] Haddock KS. Characteristics of effective discharge planning programs for the frail elderly. *J Geront Nsg.* 1991;17(7):10–14.

[16] Bull MJ. Elders' and family members' perspectives in planning for hospital discharge. *Applied Nurs Res.* 1994;7:190–192.

[17] Wertheimer DS, Kleinman LS. A model for interdisciplinary discharge planning in a university hospital. *Gerontologist.* 1990;30:837–840.

[18] Hammer BJ. Improved coordination of care for elderly patients. *Geriatr Nurs.* 1996;17(6):286–290.

[19] Sovie MD. Tailoring hospitals for managed care and integrated health systems. *Nurs Econ.* 1995;13(2):72–83.

[20] Kadushin G, Kulys R. Patient and family involvement in discharge planning. *J Geront Soc Work.* 1994;22(3/4):171–199.

[21] Moran M J, Johnson JE. Quality improvement: The nurse's role. In Dienemann J, Ed. *Continuous quality improvement in nursing.* Washington, DC: American Nurses Association; 1992:45–59.

[22] McCarthy S. The process of discharge planning. In: O'Hare P, Terry M, Eds. *Discharge planning: Strategies for assuring continuity of care.* Rockville, MD: Aspen; 1988:103–128.

[23] Naylor MD, Campbell RL, Foust JB. Meeting the discharge planning needs of hospitalized elderly and their caregivers. In Funk SG, Tornquist EM, Champagne MT, Wiese RA, Eds. *Key aspects of caring for the chronically ill.* New York: Springer Publishing Co.; 1993:142–150.

[24] Neidlinger SH, Scroggins K, Kennedy LM. Cost evaluation of discharge planning for hospitalized elderly. *Nurs Econ.* 1987;5(5):225–230.

[25] Evans RL, Hendricks RD. Evaluating hospital discharge planning: A randomized clinical trial. *Med Care.* 1993;31(4):358–370.

[26] Jackson MF. Discharge planning: Issues and challenges for gerontological nursing. A critique of the literature. *J Adv Nurs.* 1994;19:492–502.

Chapter 15

IMPLEMENTING CLINICAL PRACTICE PROTOCOLS: TRANSLATING KNOWLEDGE INTO PRACTICE

Deborah Francis, Melissa M. Bottrell, and the NICHE Faculty

Over the past 20 years, a variety of factors have converged to create the current demand for increased standardization of health care practices. The rising costs of health care, inconsistent practice patterns, adoption of new technologies by providers[1–3], and increased consumer demands have contributed to this trend toward greater standardization of medical and nursing care[4,5]. In addition, it is increasingly difficult to keep abreast of the vast amounts of research and translate that new knowledge into best practice patterns[3–5]. To meet this challenge, professional organizations and health care institutions have developed clinical practice guidelines on a wide variety of topics in an effort to improve quality of care, promote patient satisfaction, and decrease costs[2]. However, in spite of extensive protocol development and dissemination, there is pervasive evidence that the widespread availability of protocols has led neither to protocol adoption nor to desired changes in health care practice[6].

Although it may be self-evident that achieving the desired improvements in clinical care depends not only on the proper development of clinical protocols, but also on their widespread application, much of the effort in the protocol movement has focused almost exclusively on protocol development, with little attention paid to dissemination, implementation, and use[6]. Lack of attention to the process of implementation can undermine protocol adoption and derail desired changes in practice patterns. Without a clear understanding of why a protocol should be adopted, support for learning how to use it, and the belief that it will improve care, few practitioners have the desire or motivation to actually use a protocol or make changes in their clinical practice.

The first objective of this chapter is to help practitioners and institutions recognize the need to go beyond the development or modification of clinical practice protocols and concentrate on the implementation process, upon which successful adoption of protocols hinges. The chapter will highlight those factors and forces that influence clinician behavior and examine strategies that can effectively motivate clinicians to adopt innovative nursing practices, specifically the NICHE elder-focused clinical practice protocols.

HISTORY OF PROTOCOL DEVELOPMENT/ DEFINITION OF TERMS

Elder-focused clinical practice protocols, like the widely disseminated clinical practice guidelines from the Agency for Health Care Policy and Research (AHCPR), are examples of tools that are used to define how scientifically valid and reliable standards of care should be implemented. In 1973, the American Nurses Association (ANA) developed *Standards of Nursing Practice* designed to "measure the competency of nurses and evaluate the quality of nursing care"[7]. Over time, these standards acquired a patient-oriented focus emphasizing the goals of patient care. They now underpin performance improvement programs[8] and emphasize the improvement of patient outcomes through research-based interventions[7]. Clinical practice protocols, practice guidelines and algorithms, and   more recently   critical paths and care maps have emerged as tools to guide clinical nursing practice (See Table 15.1)[9]. These systematically developed statements "translate the scientific literature into concise tools intended to change clinical practice"[10] in order to improve patient outcomes and lead to more effective and efficient use of scarce medical resources.

WHY CARE ABOUT IMPLEMENTATION?

The faculty involved in the Nurses Improving Care to the Hospitalized Elderly Project (NICHE) have taken the lead to develop the best practice standards for geriatric nursing care. Developed by a panel of nationally recognized experts in geriatric nursing care, the NICHE protocols focus on assessment, prevention, and management of 14 common geriatric syndromes that contribute to functional decline in the elderly. Unlike other clinical guidelines, NICHE protocols are designed specifically to address the needs of older adults, and the interventions are primarily nurse-driven.

We recognize, however, that acceptance of a concept does not necessarily guarantee that it will be integrated into new practice patterns. Like the standards of nursing care that collect dust in hospital policy and procedure manuals between visits of the Joint Commission on Accreditation of Health Care Organizations (JCAHO), practice protocols have had limited success in changing nursing practice or improving patient outcomes. Traditional lec-

TABLE 15.1 A Protocol by Any Other Name

Procedure: Set of action steps describing how to complete a clinical function

Protocols: Precise guidelines with a structured and logical approach to a closely specified clinical problem"[37]

Standard of care: A competent level of nursing care provided to all clients as demonstrated by the nursing process"[38]

Algorithms: Set of steps that approximates the decision process of an expert clinician

Clinical Practice Guidelines: "Systematically developed statements to assist practitioner and patient decisions about appropriate health care for specific clinical circumstances"[39]

Critical Path: Multidisciplinary approach that guides the nurse in what to do when

ture-based continuing education programs are largely unsuccessful in changing provider behavior[11]. Studies have shown that distribution of guidelines to physicians through a combination of general mailings and publications, similar to what has been used by the AHCPR and other professional organizations, also do not result in desired changes in behavior[12–14]. This is one reason why the AHCPR abandoned the guideline development process, deciding instead to fund research on the critical process of implementation[4]. It has been suggested that "90% of effort needs to be in implementation," an effort that recognizes "professional, administrative and economic hurdles"[15].

A FRAMEWORK FOR IMPLEMENTATION: SOCIAL INFLUENCE THEORY

To be successful, strategies for protocol implementation must consider social influences and behavioral models of clinical decision making[6], as well as an understanding of how innovative practice is diffused among a group. The process by which "an innovation is communicated through certain channels over time among the members of a social system" is known as diffusion theory[10]. (see Figure 15.1).

This S-shaped curve demonstrates how a new idea initially is adopted by one or a few individuals, known as "innovators." In a hospital setting, they may be advanced practice nurses who believe that adoption of a protocol could improve patient care. The next group of individuals to adopt the idea are known as the "early adopters," who typically are well-respected and credible opinion leaders within the peer group. The rate of adoption of the idea takes off when the early adopters role-model and communicate best practice patterns to peers. This information sharing makes the diffusion of innovations a social process that occurs naturally as clinicians learn about the protocol, are persuaded to use it, and subsequently integrate it into practice and evaluate it for future use. Although early adopters may be easily convinced to take on a new practice, the vast majority of the group will resist change

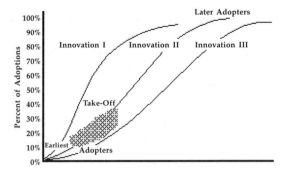

FIGURE 15.1   The S-shaped diffusion curve. This illustration of the four components of diffusion (innovation, communication channels, time, and the social system) demonstrates the take-off and the acceleration in the rate of adoption of an innovation as interpersonal networks form a critical mass of new adopters.

Reprinted with the permission of The Free Press, a Division of Simon & Schuster, Inc. *Diffusion of Innovations,* Fourth Edition by Everett M. Rogers. Copyright © 1995 by Everett M. Rogers. Copyright © 1962, 1971, 1983 by The Free Press.

until overwhelming evidence and peer pressure demonstrate that change is the only appropriate option.

Social influence theory postulates that "the behavior of one person has the effect or intention of changing how another person behaves, feels or thinks about something"[16]. This theory argues that decisions and actions are strongly guided by the habits, customs, assumptions, beliefs, and values held by peers, prevailing practice, social norms, and economic pressures[6]. As such, a colleague's judgment and beliefs about new information significantly influence how an individual nurse evaluates and uses that information.

FACTORS AFFECTING PROTOCOL ADOPTION

Successful protocol implementation will be more likely to occur if strategies address the role of social influence and the process of diffusion of ideas, while setting realistic goals for practice change. According to Greer[17], "There are no magic signatories or formulas which will cause knowledge to jump off the page into practice." To effectively motivate clinicians to integrate research-based knowledge into practice, implementers should focus attention on those factors that can facilitate or hinder the extent to which a new practice pattern is adopted by clinicians. These factors include the qualities of the protocol, characteristics of the health care professional, characteristics of the practice setting, incentives, regulation, and patient factors[18]. Although some of these factors are not amenable to change by the individual responsible for protocol implementation, highlighting and publicizing those factors that support adoption of the protocol can significantly facilitate the implementation process.

Critical attributes of a protocol that will influence the likelihood of protocol adoption and its ultimate success include its perceived advantages, complexity, compatibility with existing practices, and ease of testing and evaluating (see Table 15.2)[10]. Providers first must perceive a benefit or relative advantage to changing practice, or the protocol will be ignored. Using reliable data to identify specific problem areas and clearly articulating the significance of the problem to target staff and administrators are key steps in highlighting the need for the protocol. For instance, if staff do not recognize that a high percentage of older patients on their unit are at risk of nosocomial infection as a result of the urinary catheters placed in the emergency department, staff are unlikely to accept the necessity of an incontinence protocol.

The protocol must be clear, relatively easy to understand, and concise, containing only the most salient points. It must also be readily available to the practitioner. For example, placing the protocol in an easily accessible location on the unit, or on pocket cards with bullets or checklists, as opposed to placing it in a

TABLE 15.2   Atributes Affecting Protocol Adoption

Advantage: What benefit does the protocol provide in comparison to current practice?

Complexity: How easily can the protocol be introduced into regular practice?

Compatibility: How well does the new practice fit with the practitioner's previous experience, values, and existing beliefs?

Feasibility: How easily can the practitioner try the protocol on one patient?

Observability: Are the improvements in practice or changes readily or easily observable for the practitioner?

manual behind a desk, will encourage its use. Further, the protocol must be compatible—to the fullest possible degree—either with an individual's previous experience, or with existing beliefs and values. If a practitioner does not believe that using a behavioral approach or environmental modifications will calm an agitated patient, chemical or physical restraints will most likely remain the treatment of choice.

A good protocol must be able to be readily implemented and must easily demonstrate improvement in patient care. A protocol designed to enable nurses to identify a clinical problem and to make appropriate changes in the patient's treatment plan on their own is more likely to remain in use than one that depends on calls to other providers, or whose impact is difficult to assess. Finally, the ability of the provider to observe the protocol in practice and interact with other providers who have incorporated the new approach will facilitate its acceptance. In a review of 23 trials measuring the effectiveness of guideline dissemination on physician behavior, Grilli and Lomas validated the findings of Rogers[10] and concluded that relatively uncomplicated protocols that could be observed or tried by the clinician tended to be adopted more effectively[19].

Uncertainty about the validity or usefulness of the protocol will affect how much an individual will rely on the opinions of peers before forming a personal opinion about the protocol. The greater the uncertainty about the protocol's usefulness, the more one's attitudes and beliefs are influenced by peers[20]. Thus, attempts to implement a protocol could be hampered by an opinion leader, such as a nurse manager, who did not believe in or support the use of the protocol.

POTENTIAL BARRIERS TO PROTOCOL ADOPTION

Even with the availability of excellent protocols, modifying a health practitioner's behavior to conform to the guidelines has proven to be a difficult task and "requires complex behavioral interventions at the micro-level"[21]. Factors unrelated to the protocol may influence the ability to change practice patterns, are less easy to control for, and, if not addressed early, may undermine the implementation process. Pertinent characteristics of the health care practitioner include age, country, source of training, and knowledge of the domain that is to be addressed by the protocol. In addition, a variety of irrational forces, such as fear of change or anxiety about modifying routines even when change is perceived as desirable, can produce formidable barriers to protocol adoption. Resistance to change also can arise from an individual's psychology and life experiences, feelings of competition and jealousy, and need for rewards, autonomy, or ownership of any change out of egotism[21]. It has been suggested that nurses may harbor reservations about guidelines in general. In examining this phenomenon, Mulhall et al.[22] opined that this may be due to a prevailing perception that guidelines inherently are too rigid for the broad diversity of patients and their care needs, are not compatible with a holistic approach or the individualized nature of patient care, or undermine the way nurses perceive they work best with patients.

The characteristics of the practice setting that may hinder adoption of a practice innovation include the degree of administrative support and local constraints, such as limited resources and personnel. Commitment by nursing administration has been found to be pivotal to the use of evidence-based practice[23]. Without the commitment and support of both mid-and top-level managers, clinicians will be less apt to integrate evidence-based protocols into their practice. In a study of barriers to integrating research findings into daily practice, nurses identified 28 barriers. Eight of the top ten related to work environment and organizational processes influenced by management, including the lack of authority to change practice, insufficient time, lack of support from other staff and physicians, and management's refusal to allow implementation[24].

The prevailing culture of the institution, with its customs, attitudes, and beliefs, must actively support the protocol adoption-and-implementation process. This includes allowing the extra time required for the implementation process, and providing access to expert consultants, documentation systems and communication processes that support the new standard of care. The institutional culture must encourage the active involvement of clinicians in the process, particularly in the critical protocol review-and-modification process. Finally, once the protocol is adopted, nurse managers must hold their staff accountable for the new standard of care.

Financial or professional incentives, such as acknowledgment on performance appraisals, advancement on a clinical ladder, or provision of merit pay increases, can encourage adoption of the protocols and may be an excellent way to demonstrate institutional support for protocol use. Fear of legal liability may also affect the change process. Because protocols merely guide the nurse to meet the standard of care, adopting a protocol as a recommendation for patient care rather than an institutional policy and protocol will lessen the legal liability of the clinician[25]. Fastidious documentation, plus education and supervision of unlicensed assistive personnel, will further protect the clinician from accusations of breach of the standard of care[25]. Finally, protocols that address issues mandated by regulatory agencies will be more readily adopted, as will those dictated by patient factors such as readily observable clinical problems or consumer demands. It has been found that a restraint reduction protocol has been somewhat easier to implement in NICHE pilot sites due, in part, to the regulatory mandates of JCAHO. Effective implementation strategies need to address each of these variables in order to promote the acceptance of elder-focused protocols as the best practice standard of care for geriatric patients.

IMPLEMENTATION STRATEGIES

A variety of implementation strategies have been used in an attempt to influence provider behaviors. Because dissemination or distribution of printed material has been found to be relatively ineffective in creating desired changes in behavior, successful protocol implementation efforts rarely utilize this approach as the primary intervention strategy. More effective strategies have included active communication and attempts to identify and overcome barriers to change by using administrative and educational techniques appropriate to the specific practice setting. These secondary intervention strategies are designed to reinforce the protocol and ultimately cause providers to adopt and use it. These include educational programs and social influence strategies, such as the use of opinion leaders, audit and feedback, and academic detailing. Printed guidelines are considered secondary interventions when they serve as reference material for those already acculturated to the change process. They can also help provide interim education to new personnel as they await formal and informal instruction in the use of protocols.

In a review of the effectiveness of educational interventions, Davis and Taylor-Vaisey concluded that secondary interventions typically fall into three categories[18]. Those interventions considered to be weak because they had little impact on practitioner behavior included unsolicited mailed materials and traditional continuing medical education efforts, such as formal conferences, didactic courses, symposia, workshops, and small-group discussions. Interventions found to be moderately effective in changing clinical behavior included concurrent audit and feedback given to individual providers and delivered by peers or opinion leaders. Among the relatively strong interventions were a variety of reminder systems and academic detailing, which is defined as the influence of professional beliefs through targeted, individualized, and one-on-one education[18].

Academic detailing has been found to be very effective in changing provider prescribing patterns, although such efforts are time-consuming, costly, and affect relatively few individuals, rendering this strategy a relatively inefficient method by which to implement nursing protocols. Practice-based interventions, especially those that include patient education material, concurrent audit and feedback mechanisms, and reminders (e.g., posters and pocket cards), have also been found to be effective in adopting new practice patterns. The use of multiple interventions further increases the likelihood of an effective implementation[18].

Performance improvement efforts, such as continuous quality improvement (CQI) and workplace reengineering, constitute additional strategies used to implement protocols in an effort to improve clinical practice[26]. Because protocols aim to improve the decision making of individual practitioners, integrating the protocol adoption process into an organization's performance improvement efforts is central to making significant change. Re-engineering moves beyond CQI to examine and dramatically change core work processes in an organization, and should be considered to promote major change in those environments where change historically has been difficult to accomplish[26].

EFFECT OF SETTING ON STRATEGY: IMPLEMENTATION

The implementation strategy most effective in producing a change in behavior will vary according to the desired behavior changes, the type of practitioner, the technologies involved, and settings in which the change will occur[27]. Although designed primarily for acute care settings, the NICHE protocols can be readily modified to address the needs of older adults in other settings. Effective implementation strategies should vary, depending on the type of setting in which the protocol is introduced. Mittmann et al.[6] studied effective social-influence strategies to effect guideline implementation in three health-care settings: interpersonal settings, which include individual or small groups; moderate-sized, but cohesive groups, known as persuasion settings; and large, dispersed, or fractionated groups. Solo practitioners or small groups are amenable to an interpersonal approach. Successful strategies involve individual change agents who use one-on-one communication with one or several targeted clinicians.

In moderate-sized groups characterized by closely interacting providers, such as hospital nursing units and multispecialty physician groups practices, a strategy emphasizing the stepwise persuasion of opinion leaders, mid-level managers, then the whole staff may have the best chance of success. It is in this type of setting that the NICHE protocols are more apt to be implemented by nursing staff, and where the appropriate addressing of group norms is crucial.

Mass media is considered to be appropriate for very large provider groups or professional organizations that lack cohesion, often due to geographic dispersion. Examples of such groups are the American Nurses Association and the American Medical Association. For these groups, dissemination of information through general mailings may be the only feasible means to reach all members. Although new information is transferred at a relatively low cost per provider, the limited ability of printed material to change behavior in this setting raises doubt over its ultimate cost-effectiveness.

USING SPECIFIC SOCIAL INFLUENCE STRATEGIES TO FOSTER IMPLEMENTATION

Social influence strategies have been used successfully to implement clinical protocols in persuasion settings such as hospitals. These strategies, which include opinion leaders, performance improvement, study groups, patient care rounds and participatory guideline development, have been used to varying degrees with relative success at the various NICHE sites.

Opinion leader strategies use influential, respected individuals to model appropriate behavior and transfer new information as a means of changing clinical practice. In promoting the adoption of a NICHE protocol, opinion leaders attempt to convince colleagues that the proposed change in practice represents state-of-the-art, research-based interventions that are superior to current practice. Numerous studies in the medical literature have demonstrated the effectiveness of opinion and clinical leaders. Involvement by local physician leaders is the most crucial factor in changing physician behavior[2]. Interpersonal communication with peers is critical in influencing behavior in persuasion settings, and increased peer communication is the single most important strategy to promote the adoption of guidelines[10].

In NICHE sites, involvement of nursing opinion leaders, including outside experts, can significantly enhance protocol implementation. The support of staff members known to be excellent clinicians or a respected local nursing expert, such as a nursing school faculty member, can build both excitement about practice improvements and momentum in the implementation process. Building on this strategy, The John A. Hartford foundation recently awarded the American Geriatric Society $1.9 million in part to identify and train opinion leaders in an effort to improve clinical geriatric care. In the geriatric resource nurse (GRN) model of care, resource nurses play a crucial role as clinical opinion leaders who educate peers, model appropriate behavior, and ultimately influence changes in clinical practice[28]. Besides opinion leaders, hospitals also need to identify "organizational champions who can push the process of change forward over bureaucratic obstacles and change agents who can bring about change efficiently"[17].

Multidisciplinary performance improvement, such as CQI or total quality management (TQM), is a systematic and highly effective method of implementing new standards of care. This has the added advantage of more effectively building organizational support for institutionalization of the protocol. Convening study groups of individuals from a single discipline to examine and address a specific quality issue utilizes a less formal performance improvement process to effect change. This tactic fosters a sense of ownership in group members that makes them more apt to effectively influence one another and develop new behavioral norms. Multidisciplinary patient care rounds offer another opportunity to use social influence processes to effectively educate staff, model best practice, encourage group participation, and influence behavior. Patient care rounds are an integral component of the GRN model of care and are being used at each NICHE site to identify and more appropriately manage older patients.

Finally, participatory guideline development or review is a social influence process that involves unit-based staff to develop or critically review and modify the desired protocol. Active participation by bedside clinicians from the onset will promote a sense of ownership that has been found to be critical to the achievement of quality outcomes[29]. When staff identify and understand the need for practice change and help to design and implement the remedy, they are more likely to develop consensus and a sense of ownership, and to adopt and maintain practice changes. A sense of ownership and "action to improve" were the two key factors that determined how well quality change was accepted at the clinical level in an evaluation of implementation strategies of nursing quality systems, defined as "any specific approach or instrument that can be applied to evaluate quality"[29]. In examining both how well clinical staff accepted the system and the "perceived impact of the quality of patient care," Harvey and Kitson concluded that "bottom up ownership of quality and top led support for action and change"[29] were the most important factors. This included (1) creating a culture that encourages meaningful involvement of unit level clinical staff and promotes a sense of ownership and control, and (2) strong administrative commitment with a mechanism to provide clinicians with constructive feedback.

Although involvement of the practitioner in the implementation process is key to effective implementation, it has been found that participation, in and of itself, is insufficient to successfully change practice patterns[6]. Rather, the method used to disseminate the findings of the work group and the use of multiple intervention strategies will be more likely to enhance the effectiveness of the protocol implementation.

PROTOCOL IMPLEMENTATION PROCESS: HOW TO MAKE IT WORK

Identification of the Problem and Implementation Resources

Adoption of an innovative clinical practice will require an interactive process that focuses on improvement of processes rather than individual performance[30]. As such, performance improvement strategies can serve as an excellent vehicle to implement protocols when the protocol is identified as a solution to a clinical problem. One such model that has been used in critical care is the 10-step process to monitor and evaluate patient care developed by the JCAHO[31]. Another model is the Juran quality assurance method, which was utilized to successfully guide the implementation of a fall prevention protocol at one NICHE pilot site[32].

Regardless of the model chosen to drive the implementation of a protocol, there are four basic steps that need to be accomplished.

The institution must first recognize that a problem exists and identify that the practice protocol is the solution, then implement and institutionalize the solution[27]. If a change in nursing practice is to be adopted, the initial, essential step is to recognize that there is a discrepancy between how the institution is currently performing and how it could or should be performing[33]. This awareness of a need for change may occur within the institution, expressed by staff expectations or organizational performance data, or externally, by community or regulatory agencies. During this phase, the specific clinical problem is identified, defined, and refined. Utilization review, quality assurance, and financial data are used to identify priority areas of need. In addition, assessing the baseline knowledge and attitudes of nursing staff and identifying specific concerns related to caring for older patients will more readily clarify the problem and facilitate organizational buy-in.

Once it is recognized that the standard of care can be improved, the identification phase commences. This is the time to gather and synthesize pertinent information, develop group consensus and strategies to overcome barriers, and develop or review, critique, and modify the protocol. During this phase, a guiding philosophy of geriatric care is developed and adopted by the institution, and organizational commitment is solidified. Once the relevant protocol has been identified or drafted, interview staff to ascertain what is it they like or do not like about the protocol, and develop a screening process or criteria to identify patients who could benefit from the protocol. Patient care conferences and geriatric-specific nursing assessments via trigger cards such as the SPICES mneumonic developed by the original Geriatric Resource Nurse Model[28] are examples of screening mechanisms used in NICHE pilot sites. The SPICES card reminded staff to monitor for and address common problems of Skin breakdown, Poor nutrition, Incontinence, Confusion, Evidence of falls, and Sensory deficits and functional decline. Identification also involves reviewing institutional policies, and adapting the implementation process to meet local practice needs and situations[34]. Since protocols are guidelines that need to be individualized to each patient rather than mandated standards of care, consider how to most efficiently document those specific interventions implemented and the patient's response to them.

Implementers should also clarify whether the identified clinical problem is due to impaired decision making on the part of the providers, and/or a result of organizational systems and process problems[27]. If the problem is primarily a lack of awareness, interventions would naturally focus on identifying and effectively articulating problems through the use of performance improvement data. Knowledge deficits are best addressed through creative educational programs and unit-based social influence strategies. In settings where resistance to change is perceived to be a barrier, identify and win the support of those most resistant, provide concurrent feedback and, since nursing time is often perceived to be an issue, introduce time-management strategies. When there exists problems with organizational systems and processes, it may be more important to focus on developing and implementing a screening process to identify appropriate patients; modifying or developing documentation forms, communication processes, and patient education material; and creating reminder systems.

A multidisciplinary team of key clinical and administrative staff may be convened at either the identification or recognition phase. The team must include the right individuals who will remain committed enough to invest the time and energy critical to maintaining the momentum to complete the effort. The number and types of individuals is not as important as the person's skills, expertise, experience, and interest[35]. Staff nurses in particular need to be involved in the implementation of elder-focused protocols, since it is they who have to live with the results of the change. The organization must also provide team members with adequate support in terms of access to resources, reward systems, and any specialized training required to accomplish the task. This is also the time to identify and maximize the participation of allies, and identify and win over those individuals considered to be adversaries. Gilmore refers to this process as stakeholder mapping, in which all key stakeholders are identified and ranked according to (1) whether they are in favor of or opposed to the project, and (2) their power both within the organization and to influence the outcome of the protocol. With this information, strategies can be developed to make the most effective use of all relevant stakeholders[36].

The Implementation and Institutionalization Stages

The goal of the implementation stage is to develop a collaborative process of protocol implementation designed to ensure the actual use of the protocol by the target clinicians. The major challenge during this phase is then persuading administrators that a committee decision to adopt the protocol is just the beginning of the process—that merely placing the protocols in a unit binder will not positively impact patient care. Depending on the local environment, social influence strategies need to be considered to disseminate both printed and verbal information, educate staff, modify the medical record and information systems, develop incentives and reminders, provide concurrent feedback, and evaluate the success of the protocol. Consider using all available dissemination media: written information in newsletters and on bulletin boards, laminated pocket cards, posters, and cheat sheets, or algorithms for the unit or patient record. Routinely discuss the protocols at every opportunity, such as staff meetings, one-on-one discussions, patient-care conferences, and during shift report. Individually tailor the educational program to the target group, based on a needs assessment of knowledge deficits and attitudes, and utilize adult learning theory and creative learning strategies including sensitivity training, small-group discussions, case presentations, and a variety of media. Attention also needs to be paid to informing new employees and float nurses, since transfer of information occurs during the socialization process when an individual first encounters the new social setting[6].

A final, but critical, component of the implementation phase is the evaluation plan to monitor and evaluate the use of the protocol and provide staff with feedback to demonstrate the impact of the protocol on patient care. Continuous quality improvement and utilization review data should be considered in developing the evaluation plan. Outcome measures must address the purpose and goals of the protocol and should include both patient outcomes and staff compliance. Meaningful and constructive feedback must be provided not only to the target nursing staff, but to all staff, including other disciplines, as well as nonprofessional and temporary staff[29].

Finally, the protocol is ready to be institutionalized or integrated into the day-to-day operations of the organization. Educating new team members about the protocol and the justification for use, continuing to evaluate the outcomes, and modification of the process design will need to be considered if the protocol is to be fully integrated into nursing practice.

KEY POINTS TO REMEMBER FOR EFFECTIVE PROTOCOL IMPLEMENTATION

Kaluzny suggests that successful implementation strategies have certain core characteristics. These include:

- clarity regarding the relevant unit of analysis on the part of the implementers;
- a staged rather than a one-shot implementation;
- investment of time and energy in the development of a perceived performance gap;
- management of advocates and adversaries;
- investment in prerequisites;
- adherence to the theory of small wins;
- implementation built on existing and emerging governance mechanisms; and
- proactive management of problems and situations[26].

Institutions should be willing to assess and improve the performance of processes as opposed to individual performance. Because each stage of the implementation process possesses different challenges, it is helpful to understand exactly what stage of the process is needed in order to develop more appropriate strategies to facilitate adoption and overcome barriers. Adequate time and energy must be invested in developing a perceived performance gap and identifying barriers within the culture that will promote a strong, ongoing institutional commitment for change.

Implementation will be problematic unless the right team can be assembled and come to own the protocol, and develop among them a working alliance that is critical to tackle the day-to-day challenges of operationalizing the protocol into practice. Identify and utilize the opinion leaders, organizational leaders, and change agents, as well as those individuals who may be opposed to the plan. Enlist the efforts of committees and councils, such as CQI and peer review committees to support the protocol adoption process. Their legitimacy can facilitate the acceptance, reduce the stress on the clinical champions and perhaps discourage potential adversaries[26]. Finally, be proactive and highly visible in your endeavor. Recognize the importance of small successes in winning over additional support, publicize the attainment of small goals early on, and provide ongoing feedback to both those involved in the implementation and the decision makers. This implementation is a huge endeavor, but one that is worth every bit of the effort.

SUMMARY

Elder focused clinical practice protocols have the potential to dramatically improve patient care by fostering clinical decision-making based on best practice geriatric nursing standards. However, without an administrative commitment and a comprehensive organizational strategy, they may be perceived as unnecessary additional work for the already overburdened staff. It is critical for the organization to pay close attention to the how as well as the what of the protocols and develop highly specific, localized and targeted efforts at developing, disseminating, assimilating, evaluating and adopting geriatric patient standards of care.

REFERENCES

[1] Brook RH. Practice guidelines and practicing medicine. Are they compatible? [see comments]. *JAMA*. 1989;262:3027–3030.
[2] Wise CG, Billi JE. A model for practice guideline adaptation and implementation: Empowerment of the physician [see comments]. *Jt Comm J Qual Improv*. 1995; 21:465–476.
[3] Browman GP, Levine MN, Mohide EA, et al. The practice guidelines

development cycle: A conceptual tool for practice guidelines development and implementation. *J Clin Oncol.* 1995;13:502–512.

[4] Berg A, Atkins D, Tierney W. Clinical practice guidelines in practice and education. *J Gen Intl Med.* 1997;12:S25–S33.

[5] Jacox AK, Carr DB, Payne R. Preface: Policy issues related to clinical practice guidelines. *J Pain Symptom Manage.* 1994;9:143–145.

[6] Mittman BS, Tonesk X, Jacobson PD. Implementing clinical practice guidelines: Social influence strategies and practitioner behavior change. *Quarterly Review Bulletin.* 1992:413–422.

[7] Schumacher SB. Integrating guidelines into nursing practice. *Medsurg Nurs.* 1996;5:366,374–377.

[8] Mize CP, Bentley G, Hubbard S. Standards of care: Integrating nursing care plans and quality assurance activities. *AACN Clin Issues Crit Care Nurs.* 1991;2:63–68.

[9] Dracup K. Putting clinical practice guidelines to work. *Nursing.* 1996;26:41–44,46;quiz 47.

[10] Rogers EM. Lessons for guidelines from the diffusion of innovations. *Jt Comm J Qual Improv.* 1995;21:324–328.

[11] Davis DA, Thomson MA, Oxman AD, Haynes RB. Changing physician performance. A systematic review of the effect of continuing medical education strategies [see comments]. *JAMA.* 1995;274:700–705.

[12] Oxman AD, Thomson MA, Davis DA, Haynes RB. No magic bullets: A systematic review of 102 trials of interventions to improve professional practice. *CMAJ.* 1995;153:1423–1431.

[13] Lomas J, Anderson GM, Domnick-Pierre K, Vayda E, Enkin MW, Hannah WJ. Do practice guidelines guide practice? The effect of a consensus statement on the practice of physicians. *N Engl J Med.* 1989;321:1306–1311.

[14] Weingarten S, Stone E, Hayward R, et al. The adoption of preventive care practice guidelines by primary care physicians: do actions match intentions? *J Gen Intern Med.* 1995;10:138–144.

[15] McNeil C. Clinical guidelines: implementing them won't be easy [news]. *J Natl Cancer Inst.* 1996;88:488–490.

[16] Zimbardo PG, Leippe MR. *The Psychology of Attitude Change and Social Influence.* Philadelphia: Temple University Press; 1991.

[17] Greer AL. The state of the art versus the state of the science. The diffusion of new medical technologies into practice. *Int J Technol Assess Health Care.* 1988;4:5–26.

[18] Davis DA, Taylor-Vaisey A. Translating guidelines into practice: A systematic review of theoretic concepts, practical experience and

research evidence in the adoption of clinical practice guidelines [see comments]. *Cmaj.* 1997;157:408–416.

[19] Grilli R, Lomas J. Evaluating the message: The relationship between compliance rate and the subject of a practice guideline. *Med Care.* 1994;32:202–213.

[20] Bandura A. *Social foundations of thought and action: A social cognitive theory.* Englewood Cliffs, NJ: Prentice-Hall; 1986.

[21] Backer TE. Integrating behavioral and systems strategies to change clinical practice. *Jt Comm J Qual Improv.* 1995;21:351–353.

[22] Mulhall A, Alexander C, Le May A. Prescriptive care? Guidelines and protocols. *Nurs Stand.* 1997;11:43–46.

[23] Champion VL, Leach A. Variables related to research utilization in nursing: An empirical investigation. *J Adv Nurs.* 14, 1989:705–710.

[24] Funk SG, Tornquist EM, Champagne MT. Barriers and facilitators of research utilization. An integrative review. *Nurs Clin North Am.* 1995;30:395–407.

[25] Murphy RN. Legal and practical impact of clinical practice guidelines on nursing and medical practice. *Nurse Pract.* 1997;22:138,147–148.

[26] Kaluzny AD, Konrad TR, McLaughlin CP. Organizational strategies for implementing clinical guidelines [see comments]. *Jt Comm J Qual Improv.* 1995;21:347–351.

[27] Kibbe DC, Kaluzny AD, McLaughlin CP. Integrating guidelines with continuous quality improvement: Doing the right thing the right way to achieve the right goals. *Jt Comm J Qual Improv.* 1994;20:181–191.

[28] Fulmer TT. Grow your own experts in hospital elder care. *Geriatr Nurs.* 1991;12:64–66.

[29] Harvey G, Kitson A. Achieving improvement through quality: An evaluation of key factors in the implementation process. *J Adv Nurs.* 1996;24:185–195.

[30] James BC. Implementing practice guidelines through clinical quality improvement [see comments]. *Front Health Serv Manage.* 1993;10:3–37;discussion 54–56.

[31] Walker J, Claflin N. Standards of care and practice: a vital link in quality assurance. *AACN Clin Issues Crit Care Nurs.* 1991;2:90–95.

[32] Juran JM, Gryna FM, Jr. *Quality Control Handbook.* New York: McGraw-Hill; 1974.

[33] Kaluzny A, McLaughlin C, Kibbe D. Continuous quality improvement in the clinical setting: Enhancing adoption. *Qual Mgmt Hlth Care.* 1992;1:37–44.

[34] Gates P. Think globally, act locally: An approach to implementation of clinical practice guidelines. *J Qual Impt.* 1995;21:71–84.

[35] NICHE. A planning and implementation guide. Nurses Improving Care to the Hospitalized Elderly. New York University Division of Nursing, New York: Nurses Improving Care to the Hospitalized Elderly; 1997.

[36] Gilmore T. *Making a Leadership Change: How Organizations and Leaders Can Handle Leadership Change Successfully.* San Francisco: Jossey-Bass; 1988.

[37] Jenkins D. Investigations. How to get from guidelines to protocols. *Br Med J.* 1991;303:323–333.

[38] American Nurses Association. *Standards of clinical nursing practice.* Kansas City, MO; 1991.

[39] Woolf, SH. Practice guidelines: A new reality in medicine. 1. Recent developments. *Arch Intern Med.* 1990;150:1811–1818.

INDEX

INDEX

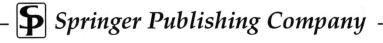
Springer Publishing Company

Restraint-Free Care
A Guide for Individualized Clinical Practice

Neville E. Strumpf, PhD, RN, C, FAAN
Joanne E. Patterson, PhD, RN
Joan Stockman Wagner, MSN, CRNP
Lois K. Evans, DNSc, RN, FAAN

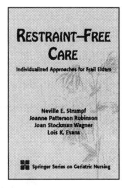

This book is for individuals seeking information on restraint-free care. Organized in outline format, the authors highlight critical material to be readily adaptable as a quick reference for clinicians, or as an adjunct for teaching staff, educating administrators, board members, and consumers.

A philosophy of individualized care is the framework for this guide, which the authors believe to be key to understanding older adults and to providing restraint-free care. The goals of individualized care include promoting comfort and safety, optimizing function and independence, and achieving the greatest possible quality of life. Such care requires clinicians to make sense of behavior rather than to control responses of clients.

The book contains specific strategies of understanding behavior; effecting change for the individual, the environment and institution; managing the risk of falls; and interference with recent treatments. Case studies and lists of resources are included in this practical and information-packed resource.

Contents: Preface • Rethinking Restraint Use • Implementing a Process of Change • Making Sense of Behavior • Responding to Behavioral Phenomena • Assessment and Prevention of Falls and Injurious Falls • Caring for the Person Who Interferes with Treatment • Maintaining a Process of Change

1998   168pp   0-8261-1215-3   softcover

536 Broadway, New York, NY 10012-3955 • (212) 431-4370 • Fax (212) 941-7842

Springer Publishing Company

Geriatric Interdisciplinary Team Training

Eugenia L. Siegler, MD, FACP,
Kathy Hyer, DrPA, MPP
Terry Fulmer, RN, PhD, FAAN,
Mathy Mezey, RN, EdD, FAAN
Editors

Geriatric
Interdisciplinary
Team Training

Eugenia L. Siegler,
Kathryn Hyer,
Terry Fulmer,
Mathy Mezey
Editors

Springer Publishing Company

"This book provides a robust analysis of the critical issues relevant to the next phase of geriatric interdisciplinary team training in the United States. It is a critical resource...."
—from the foreword by **John W. Rowe**, M.D.

The authors discuss their experience as participants in the groundbreaking Hartford Foundation initiative to create geriatric interdisciplinary team training (GITT) programs in eight model sites nationwide. They suggest various solutions to the problems encountered while designing and implementing GITT programs. Creative initiative and energetic cooperation from the authors will inspire readers to pursue similar training venues in geriatric care.

Partial Contents:

A Perspective on Health Care Teams and Team Training, *R.A. Tsukuda* • Recruiting Students for GITT, *S. Moore* • Selecting and Preparing Team Training Educators, *E.R. Mackenzie et al.* • Using Existing and Emerging Technologies to Promote GITT, *S. Levkoff, P.F. Weitzman, E.A. Weitzman* • Structuring the GITT Didactic Experience, *J.L. Howe, C.K. Cassel, M. Vezina* • Structuring the GITT Clinical Experience, *J. Farness, V. Fay, A. Schneider, N. Wilson, M. Gleason* • Evaluating the Effects of GITT, *T. Fulmer and K. Hyer* • Geriatric Team Training in Managed Care Organizations, *J. Frank and R. Della Penna* • Turning the Clinical Agency into a Setting for Team Training: The On Lok Experience, *K. O'Malley, S. Kornblatt, and C. Van Steenberg*

1998   304pp   0-8261-1210-2   hardcover

536 Broadway, New York, NY 10012-3955 • (212) 431-4370 • Fax (212) 941-7842